Essentials of Neuroimaging for Clinical Practice

Edited by

Darin D. Dougherty, M.D., M.Sc.

Scott L. Rauch, M.D.

Jerrold F. Rosenbaum, M.D.

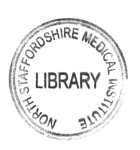

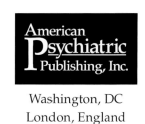

American **Psychiatric** Publishing, Inc.

Washington, DC
London, England

Note: The authors have worked to ensure that all information in this book is accurate at the time of publication and consistent with general psychiatric and medical standards, and that information concerning drug dosages, schedules, and routes of administration is accurate at the time of publication and consistent with standards set by the U.S. Food and Drug Administration and the general medical community. As medical research and practice continue to advance, however, therapeutic standards may change. Moreover, specific situations may require a specific therapeutic response not included in this book. For these reasons and because human and mechanical errors sometimes occur, we recommend that readers follow the advice of physicians directly involved in their care or the care of a member of their family.

Copyright © 2004 American Psychiatric Publishing, Inc.
ALL RIGHTS RESERVED

Manufactured in the United States of America on acid-free paper
08 07 06 05 04   5 4 3 2 1
First Edition

Typeset in Adobe's Palatino and Futura Book

American Psychiatric Publishing, Inc.
1000 Wilson Boulevard
Arlington, VA 22209–3901
www.appi.org

Library of Congress Cataloging-in-Publication Data
Essentials of neuroimaging for clinical practice / edited by Darin D. Dougherty, Scott L. Rauch, Jerrold F.
    Rosenbaum
        p. ; cm.
    Includes bibliographical references and index.
    ISBN 1-58562-079-3 (alk. paper)
    1. Brain—Imaging. I. Dougherty, Darin D. II. Rauch, Scott L. III. Rosenbaum, J. F. (Jerrold F.)
    [DNLM: 1. Diagnostic Imaging. 2. Mental Disorders—diagnosis. WM 141 E78 2003]
    RC386.6.D52E84 2003
    616.8′04754—dc21   2003052221

British Library Cataloguing in Publication Data
A CIP record is available from the British Library.

About the cover:
Top (left and right): Effect of image acquisition parameters on functional magnetic resonance imaging (fMRI) signal. *Middle:* Color-coded diffusion tensor imaging (DTI): Anisotropy *(left)* and color-coded DTI *(right)* of a healthy control subject. *Source.* Reprinted from Taber KH, Pierpaoli C, Rose SE, et al.: "The Future for Diffusion Tensor Imaging in Neuropsychiatry." *Journal of Neuropsychiatry and Clinical Neurosciences* 14:1–5, 2002. Copyright 2002. Used with permission.
Bottom left: Acute embolic stroke on computed tomography (CT) (hypodense lesion indicated by arrow).
Bottom right: 15-Oxygen positron emission tomography (^{15}O PET) data acquired from a patient during an acute ischemic event.

To my wife,
Christina,
and our children,
Emma and William

D.D.D.

To my family,
for all of their support

S.L.R.

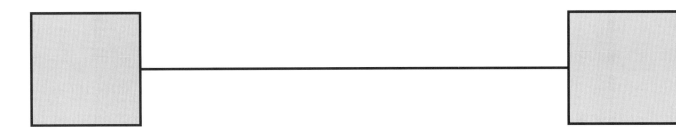

Contents

Lawrence T. Park, M.D.
Ramon Gilberto Gonzalez, M.D.

Martin A. Goldstein, M.D.
Bruce H. Price, M.D.

Darin D. Dougherty, M.D., M.Sc.
Scott L. Rauch, M.D.
Alan J. Fischman, M.D., Ph.D.

Robert L. Savoy, Ph.D.
Randy L. Gollub, M.D., Ph.D.

List of Tables

List of Illustrations

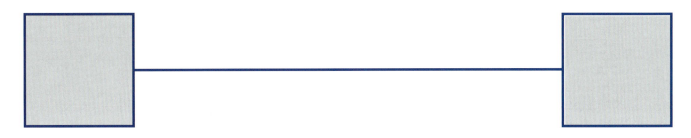

Contributors

Nicolas Bolo, Ph.D.
Associate Biophysicist, Brain Imaging Center; Lecturer in Psychiatry, McLean Hospital, Harvard Medical School, Belmont, Massachusetts

Darin D. Dougherty, M.D., M.Sc.
Assistant Director of Psychiatric Neuroimaging Research, Departments of Psychiatry and Radiology, Massachusetts General Hospital; Assistant Professor of Psychiatry, Harvard Medical School, Boston, Massachusetts

Alan J. Fischman, M.D., Ph.D.
Director, Department of Nuclear Medicine, Massachusetts General Hospital; Professor of Radiology, Harvard Medical School, Boston, Massachusetts

Martin A. Goldstein, M.D.
Instructor of Neurology, Weill Medical College, Cornell University, New York, New York

Randy L. Gollub, M.D., Ph.D.
Assistant Director of Psychiatric Neuroimaging Research, Departments of Psychiatry and Radiology, Massachusetts General Hospital; Assistant Professor of Psychiatry, Harvard Medical School, Boston, Massachusetts

Ramon Gilberto Gonzalez, M.D.
Director of Neuroradiology, Massachusetts General Hospital; Associate Professor of Radiology, Harvard Medical School, Boston, Massachusetts

Gina R. Kuperberg, M.D., Ph.D.
Psychiatrist, Department of Psychiatry, Massachusetts General Hospital; Assistant Professor of Psychiatry, Harvard Medical School, Boston, Massachusetts

Lawrence T. Park, M.D.
Director, Acute Psychiatry Service, Massachusetts General Hospital; Instructor in Psychiatry, Harvard Medical School, Boston, Massachusetts

Bruce H. Price, M.D.
Assistant Professor of Neurology, Harvard Medical School, Boston, Massachusetts; Chief, Department of Neurology, McLean Hospital, Belmont, Massachusetts

Scott L. Rauch, M.D.
Associate Chief of Psychiatry for Neuroscience Research and Director of Psychiatric Neuroimaging Research, Departments of Psychiatry and Radiology, Massachusetts General Hospital; Associate Professor of Psychiatry, Harvard Medical School, Boston, Massachusetts

Perry F. Renshaw, M.D., Ph.D.
Director, Brain Imaging Center, and Associate Professor, McLean Hospital, Harvard Medical School, Belmont, Massachusetts

Jerrold F. Rosenbaum, M.D.
Chief of Psychiatry, Massachusetts General Hospital; Professor of Psychiatry, Harvard Medical School

Robert L. Savoy, Ph.D.
Senior Scientist, The Athinoula A. Martinos Center for Biomedical Imaging, Charlestown, Massachusetts

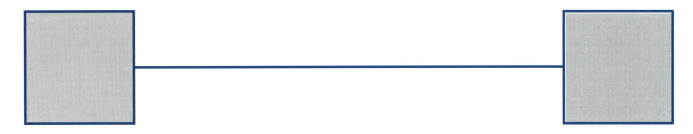

Introduction

Neuroimaging technology has progressed considerably during recent decades. Neuroimaging studies can be an invaluable part of the diagnostic workup of psychiatric patients. However, it can be difficult to determine which clinical situations call for the use of neuroimaging studies and which do not. In addition, it is often unclear what type of neuroimaging study should be ordered. Should contrast be used during the study? Are there specific acquisition parameters that may be useful in a particular clinical situation? The goal of this volume is to describe the currently available neuroimaging technologies and to discuss their appropriate use in the clinical psychiatric setting. The potential future clinical utility of these techniques will be addressed as well.

Structural neuroimaging modalities such as computed tomography (CT) and magnetic resonance imaging (MRI) have revolutionized the practice of medicine in recent decades. In the first chapter, **Park and Gonzalez** describe the history of CT, how CT works, and which clinical situations call for the use of CT. The chapter also provides a number of CT images as examples of radiological findings associated with specific diagnoses. **Goldstein and Price** present similar detail in their chapter on MRI. This chapter summarizes the state of the art in MRI technology and offers specific guidelines for ordering MRI studies.

Functional neuroimaging techniques developed after the advent of structural neuroimaging and show great promise for both clinical use and neuroscience research. Positron emission tomography (PET) and single photon emission computed tomography (SPECT) have demonstrated the greatest clinical utility of all functional neuroimaging methods to date. The chapter by **Dougherty, Rauch, and Fischman** reviews the physics underlying PET and SPECT and highlights the usefulness of these technologies in clinical situations. Functional magnetic resonance imaging (fMRI) has limited clinical utility in psychiatry at present, but it is a powerful tool that shows great potential for future application. **Savoy and Gollub** provide an understandable and lucid description of fMRI and discuss possible future clinical uses. Magnetic resonance spectroscopy (MRS) is another technology that uses unique MRI acquisition parameters to assess in vivo brain neurochemistry. **Bolo and Renshaw** delineate the current capabilities of MRS and consider future potential uses.

Electroencephalography (EEG) has been used for almost a century to measure cortical electrical activity. **Kuperberg** outlines recent developments in the EEG field, including quantitative EEG and event-related potentials. This chapter also describes a related technology, magnetoencephalography.

Finally, **Rauch** offers a perspective on the future of neuroimaging in psychiatric practice as well as in research. This chapter clearly characterizes the tremendous potential that these methods hold for advances in our field.

Acknowledgments

We would like to acknowledge our mentors and collaborators; in particular, we wish to express our appreciation to Michael A. Jenike, M.D., Nathaniel M. Alpert, Ph.D., Alan J. Fischman, M.D., Ph.D., Robert H. Rubin, M.D., and Ned Cassem, M.D. Finally, we wish to thank the editorial and production staff of American Psychiatric Publishing, Inc., for their expertise, support, and patience.

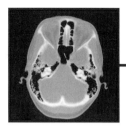

Computed Tomography

Lawrence T. Park, M.D.
Ramon Gilberto Gonzalez, M.D.

Computed tomography (CT), or computerized axial tomography (CAT), was one of the first noninvasive imaging techniques for three-dimensional (3D) visualization of neuroanatomic structure. Before CT, the main modes of imaging cerebral structure, ventriculography and pneumoencephalography, relied on plain-film technology and were quite invasive. The advent of CT revolutionized the field of neuropsychiatry and ushered in a new era of neuroimaging. CT provided a tool to create reliable and accurate representations of internal structure using noninvasive techniques and, as a result, fostered an acceleration in the growth of the neurosciences (as well as other medical fields). Despite the development of other imaging technologies (such as magnetic resonance imaging [MRI]), CT continues to play an important role in the practice of clinical neuropsychiatry. CT offers distinct advantages over other imaging modalities. CT provides excellent image quality and rapid acquisition time at relatively low cost. Moreover, CT is widely available, with approximately 75% of all U.S. hospitals having access to CT. In many clinical situations, CT remains the diagnostic study of first choice. In this chapter we examine the history and development of CT, technical aspects of CT imaging, nor-mal and abnormal findings in CT imaging, and clinical indications for neuroimaging in general, and we offer guidance for selecting between CT and MRI.

History and Development

The first CT images were produced in the late 1960s by Sir Godfrey Hounsfield of Electro-Musical Instruments (EMI) Limited. Hounsfield, an engineer with the British music label, elaborated concepts underlying CT imaging and created the technology necessary to collect the needed data for imaging. Following principles of image reconstruction described by Radon in the early 1900s and tissue attenuation principles initially set forth by Cormack in the 1950s, Hounsfield proposed theories that supported the possibility of assessing internal structure through a series of X-ray transmissions and measurements around the periphery of a body (Figure 1–1). From these principles, Hounsfield constructed the first CT scanner and, for his groundbreaking work, received the Nobel Prize in Medicine in 1979 (with Cormack). The first scans acquired 28,800 inde-

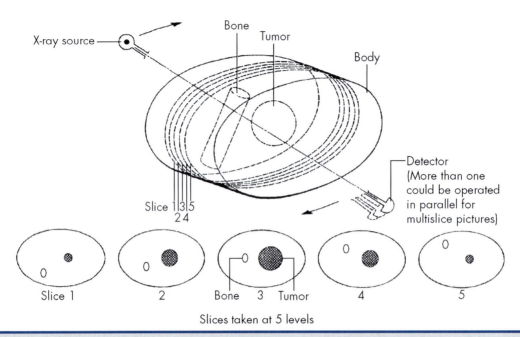

Figure 1–1. CT data acquisition techniques: rotating source and detector around a body.
Source. Reprinted from Hounsfield GN: "Computerized Transverse Axial Scanning (Tomography), Part I: Description of System." *British Journal of Radiology* 46:1016–1022, 1973. Copyright 1973, British Institute of Radiology. Used with permission.

pendent measurements, requiring 9 hours of acquisition time. The final image consisted of an 80×80 matrix (6,400 voxels), which took 9 days to reconstruct from the initial measurements (Figure 1–2). The first commercially available machines were produced in 1973 by EMI; these were capable of reconstructing an 80×80–voxel image in 10 minutes.

Since that time, CT technology has advanced significantly, providing higher-resolution images and faster scanning times. Current high-speed (helical, spiral, or multidetector) scanners can acquire data for full-body imaging in less than 3 minutes and provide images with spatial resolution of less than 1 square millimeter. In addition, other CT-based technologies have been developed (Table 1–1). CT angiography and other 3D reconstruction techniques have been developed and offer high-resolution 3D representations of vascular (or other anatomic) structure. CT myelography remains a valuable technique for evaluating the spinal cord and related structures. Single photon emission computed tomography (SPECT; see Chapter 3 in this volume) provides functional representations of cerebral physiology and, like other functional imaging techniques (e.g., positron emission tomography [PET]; see Chapter 3), is based on common imaging principles that make use of radioactive markers paired with physiological correlates of function to provide functional representations of cerebral physiology.

Table 1–1. CT–based imaging technologies

High-speed multidetector CT
Three-dimensional reconstruction
CT angiography
CT myelography
Single photon emission CT (SPECT)

Technical Considerations

CT uses essentially the same basic technology as plain-film X rays. In plain-film radiography, an X-ray source transmits gamma rays through a part of the body, and a detector (e.g., the film) on the other side measures the amount of radiation not absorbed by the body. As the X rays pass through the body, different tissues absorb radiation in varying degrees (X-ray absorption is generally related to electron density of the tissue). For example, in a plain film of the chest, X rays pass through different structures of the thorax. When X rays pass through denser structures such as bone, relatively more radiation is absorbed (i.e., there is greater attenuation of the initial X-ray transmission), resulting in less exposure of the film on the other side of the chest. Less exposure of the film corresponds to a bright (or white) representation on the film. When X rays pass through lung tissue (a less dense

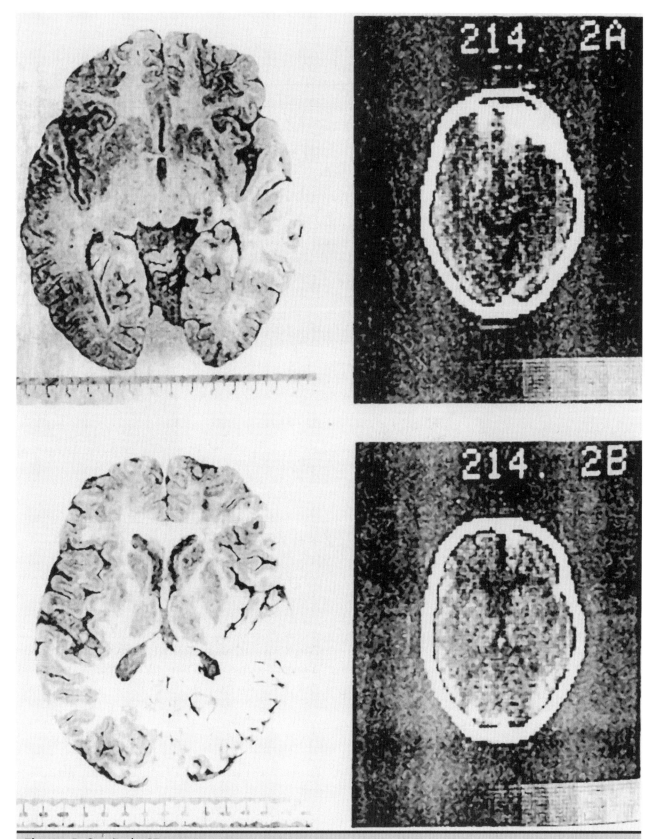

Figure 1–2. Early CT imaging.

A, Horizontal sections of normal human brain. **B,** Early CT images at the corresponding transverse plane.

Source. Reprinted from Ambrose J: "Computerized Transverse Axial Scanning (Tomography), Part 2: Clinical Application." *British Journal of Radiology* 46:1023–1047, 1973. Copyright 1973, British Institute of Radiology. Used with permission.

tissue), relatively less radiation is absorbed, leading to greater exposure of the film and a darker (or black) image. When X rays pass through heart tissue or muscle (intermediate density), there is intermediate absorption, and the resulting image is an intermediate one (shade of gray).

The plain radiographic film represents equally all structures through which X rays pass and superimposes all images on a two-dimensional surface (the film itself). In contrast, whereas a tomogram makes use of the same basic method of X-ray transmission, the resulting image is focused in a specific plane of the body through which the X rays traversed. Tomograms provide the sharpest images in that one plane, with superimposed blurred images of structures lying on either side of that plane.

CT scanning consists of a series of tomograms, or slices, through sections of the body. However, its method of image acquisition differs from that used in conventional tomography. In CT, instead of transmitting X rays perpendicularly through the body and then taking measurements in a focused plane with conventional radiological film, a series of transmissions and measurements are performed around the periphery of a body. Rotating around a body, X rays are transmitted by an X-ray emitter, pass through the body, and are measured by a detector on the opposite side. Measurement is accomplished with a paired X-ray source and detector positioned 180 degrees from each other. This apparatus rotates around one plane of the head, and

X-ray attenuation is measured at multiple points throughout a 360-degree arc around the body (Figure 1–3, A and B). By means of computer-assisted algorithms, an image of the somatic structure within the slice is constructed from the multiple measurements taken around the body. The slice through which the X rays traverse is separated into a grid, with each box in the grid (voxel or pixel) representing a small area of the body. By analyzing the X-ray attenuation of each of the data points around the body, an attenuation value for each voxel within the body may be calculated. Each voxel is assigned an attenuation value from +500 to –500 (called *Hounsfield units*). By convention, water is assigned a value of zero (Figure 1–4). The representation of the attenuation for all the voxels of the grid produces a structural image within that plane.

The use of intravenous radio-opaque contrast significantly improves the ability of CT to visualize certain normal and abnormal structures. Contrast highlights vascular structures as well as lesions that lead to compromise of the blood–brain barrier. As a result, vascular abnormalities such as aneurysms, dissections, and arteriovenous malformations will be more easily visualized (although angiography remains the study of choice when these lesions are suspected). Contrast will also highlight lesions that lead to gross disruption of the blood–brain barrier. Such lesions include inflammatory processes of the brain (e.g., infection) and tumors (Table 1–2).

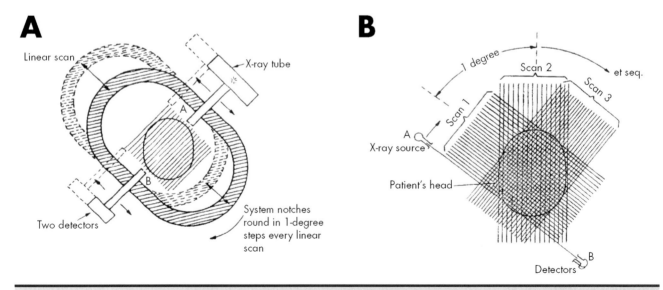

Figure 1–3. CT image acquisition.
A, Motion of frame and detectors for producing two continuous slices. **B,** Illustration of scanning sequence.
Source. Reprinted from Hounsfield GN: "Computerized Transverse Axial Scanning (Tomography), Part 1: Description of System." *British Journal of Radiology* 46:1016–1022, 1973. Copyright 1973, British Institute of Radiology. Used with permission.

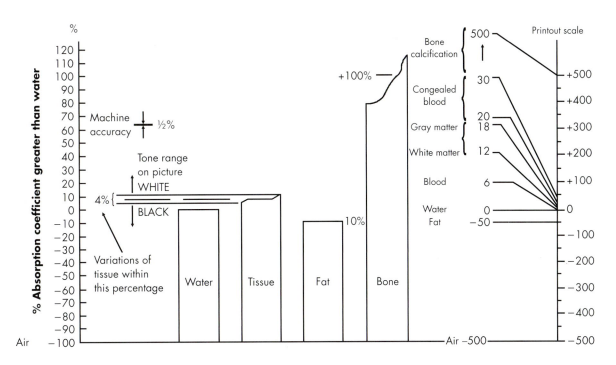

Density	Tissue	Hounsfield units	Visual representation
High	Mineral/bone	+1 to +500	White
Medium	Water/fluid	0	Gray
Low	Air/lung	–1 to –500	Black

Figure 1–4. Attenuation values of various tissue types: Hounsfield units.
Illustration of machine sensitivity. The scale on the right is an arbitrary scale used on the printout and is related to water=0, air=–500 units. It can be seen that most materials to be detected fall within 20 units above zero and can be covered by the adjustable 4% "window."
Source. Reprinted from Hounsfield GN: "Computerized Transverse Axial Scanning (Tomography): Part 1. Description of System." *British Journal of Radiology* 46:1016–1022, 1973. Copyright 1973, British Institute of Radiology. Used with permission.

Table 1–2. Indications for use of intravenous contrast with specific lesions

Intravenous contrast study indicated

Aneurysms

Dissections

Inflammatory processes of meninges

Infection/abscess

Tumors

Noncontrast study indicated

Acute or unstable situations

Hemorrhage

Hydrocephalus

Cerebral edema

Fractures

Pneumocephalus

Calcifications

Metal/foreign body

Two types of contrast material are currently in use: ionic and non-ionic. Ionic contrast is manufactured from iodinated compounds and is high in osmolarity. Ionic contrast is more commonly used and comparatively less expensive than non-ionic contrast and is generally indicated unless there is a history of adverse reaction. Non-ionic contrast, which is less allergenic, is manufactured from low-osmolarity compounds such as iohexol or iopamidol and is significantly more expensive.

Adverse reactions to ionic contrast include chemotoxic reactions and idiosyncratic reactions. Chemotoxic reactions may affect the brain or kidneys. Chemotoxic reactions of the brain manifest as an increased risk of seizures. The baseline risk of seizures with ionic contrast administration is 1 in 10,000 if the blood–brain barrier is intact and slightly higher if the blood–brain barrier is compromised. Chemotoxic reactions may also affect the kidneys and may lead to renal dysfunction (from azotemia to renal failure). There is a 1% risk

Table 1–3.   Risk factors for adverse reaction to ionic contrast

Previous adverse reaction to ionic contrast
Creatinine level >2.0 mg/dL
History of diabetes mellitus
Age <1 year
Age >60 years
History of asthma
History of allergies

of decreased renal function with ionic contrast administration in patients with normal serum creatinine levels (<1.5 mg/dL). However, the risk increases to approximately one-third for those with a serum creatinine level greater than 4.5 mg/dL. The risk of renal dysfunction is also higher for individuals with a history of diabetes mellitus. Idiosyncratic reactions may also occur in up to 5% of patients receiving ionic contrast. Symptoms include hypotension, nausea, flushing, rash, urticaria, and anaphylaxis. Risk factors for idiosyncratic reactions include age less than 1 year, age greater than 60

years, history of asthma, significant history of allergies, and past adverse reaction to ionic contrast (Table 1–3). As a rule of thumb, a known history of ionic contrast reaction, a creatinine level greater than 2.0 mg/dL, or the presence of active renal failure serve as contraindications to administration of ionic contrast. In these cases, non-ionic contrast should be considered the medium of choice.

Normal and Abnormal Findings

A typical CT scan of the head consists of a *scout view* (similar to a plain film X ray in coronal and/or sagittal section) and a series of transverse tomograms (Figure 1–5). One can vary the width of the slice, as well as the distance between slices. In addition, by varying the acquisition parameters, different visualization techniques can allow for more sensitive assessment of certain types of tissue. For example, *brain windows* provide

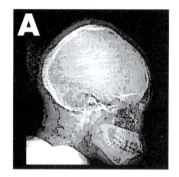

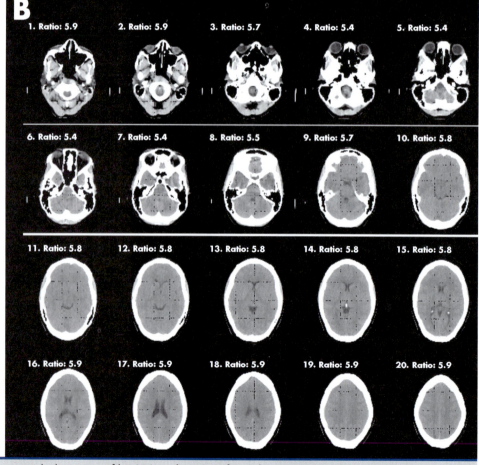

Figure 1–5.   Typical CT scan, including scout film **(A)** and series of axial tomograms **(B)**.

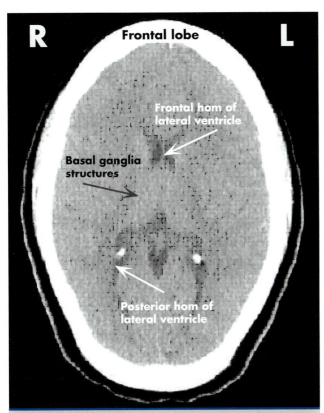

Figure 1–6. CT scan showing transverse view of normal brain at the level of the basal ganglia. *Arrows* demonstrate the frontal and posterior horns of the lateral ventricle.

optimal visualization of brain tissue, whereas *bone windows* provide optimal visualization of bony structures. CT bone windows are the best imaging technique for assessing the integrity of the cortical bone structure; CT brain windows provide optimal viewing of brain parenchyma and vascular structure.

CT generally provides excellent visualization of normal structures of the brain. Figure 1–6 demonstrates a transverse view of a normal brain at the level of the frontal horns of the lateral ventricle. In the CT image, there is excellent visualization of the cortical bone structure as well as the ventricular system. Bone in these images is seen as bright (white). The cerebrospinal fluid (CSF)–filled ventricular system is dark (black). The brain parenchyma is well visualized, although there is limited differentiation between gray and white matter. Gray matter is seen as lighter gray, whereas white matter, being less dense, appears slightly darker. In Figure 1–7, brain and bone windows are represented. Taken from the level of the base of the skull, these images demonstrate the optic structures, sinuses, mastoid air cells, and other otic structures. The bone windows high-

light these structures. The brain windows provide better visualization of the parenchymal structures. At this level, one can observe the limited visualization of the cerebellum and brain stem due to streaks (artifact) produced by the thick surrounding bone.

Pathology that is best visualized by CT includes acute hemorrhage (particularly subarachnoid hemorrhage), calcified lesions, and certain types of bony lesions. Bony lesions well visualized by CT include fractures (Figure 1–8) and lytic (or blastic) lesions. Single lytic lesions may represent a single meningioma, hemangioma, or metastasis. Multiple lytic lesions may represent Paget's disease, multiple myeloma, or multiple metastases.

Subdural hematoma typically appears as a crescentic lesion between the skull and brain (Figure 1–9). Depending on the temporal aspects of the lesions, subdural hematoma lesions may appear differently. In the acute setting (less than 1 week), hematomas characteristically appear as high-density (bright) lesions. As the hematoma evolves over time, the lesion becomes progressively less dense. In the subacute setting (1 week to several weeks), the lesion appears as isodense (gray). In the chronic setting (over a period of months), the lesion may appear as hypodense (dark) or may be reabsorbed, leaving a cavity in the space once occupied by the hematoma. The temporal evolution of the appearance of blood on CT is presented in Table 1–4.

Epidural hematoma is typically seen as a rapidly developing, high-density (bright) biconvex lesion between the skull and brain, which often displaces cortical matter (Figure 1–10). The majority of epidural hematomas occur as a result of traumatic dissection of a branch of the middle meningeal artery, and associated findings may include temporal bone fracture. Subarachnoid hemorrhage appears as a thin line of high-density (bright) signal that outlines the area between the surface of the brain and regions of CSF (e.g., sulci, fissures, basal cistern) (Figure 1–11). CT (with contrast) is quite sensitive for acute subarachnoid hemorrhage and remains an important tool for its initial detection. In contrast to subdural hematoma, subarachnoid hemorrhage may evolve relatively quickly over time and may not be visible by CT several days after the initial hemorrhage.

Contusions are often seen as hypodense (dark) lesions within the brain parenchyma. They are frequently located in frontal or temporal lobes and are typically caused by traumatic injury in that area (Figure 1–12). Contracoup contusions may be seen as hypodense lesions located on the opposite side of traumatic

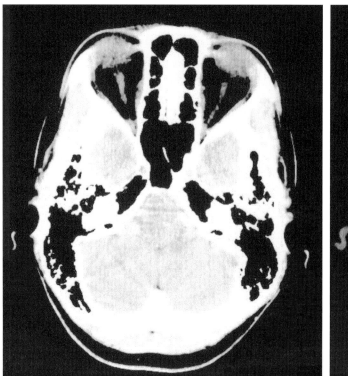
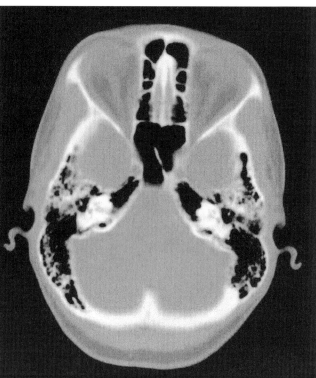

Figure 1–7.   CT scan of a normal brain: brain and bone windows at the level of the mastoid air cells.

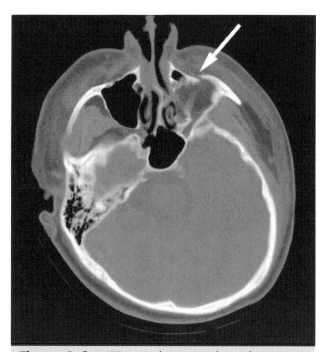

Figure 1–8.   CT scan: bone windows demonstrating a facial fracture.

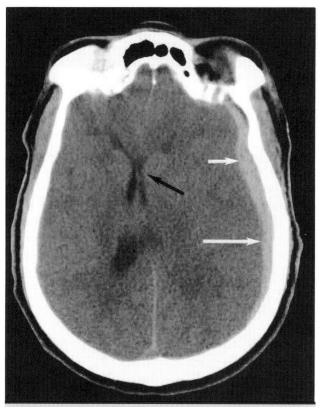

Figure 1–9.   Subdural hematoma, subacute phase. Hematoma indicated by *white arrows*; mass effect indicated by *black arrow*.

Table 1-4. Temporal evolution of blood on CT

Setting	Time	Density	Appearance	Other
Acute	Less than 1 week	Hyperdense	Bright	
Subacute	Up to several weeks	Isodense	Gray	
Chronic	More than several weeks	Hypodense	Dark	Blood may reabsorb

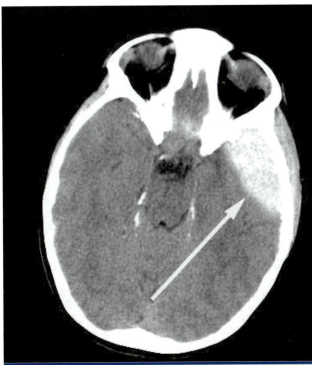

Figure 1-10. Epidural hematoma, acute, with contrast.

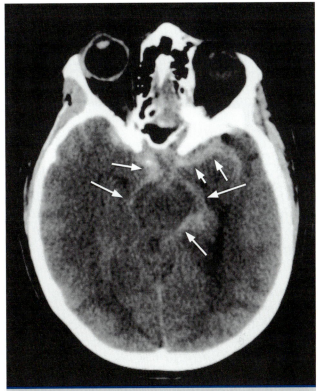

Figure 1-11. Subarachnoid hemorrhage, acute. Thin bright line highlighted with *arrows* represents bleeding.

injury (e.g., occipital lesion in association with frontal/temporal injury).

CT is also useful for the evaluation of stroke. In fact, because of its widespread availability and speed, CT is the initial diagnostic study of choice in many stroke protocols. In the acute setting, if thrombolytic therapy is being considered for an embolic event, CT is nearly as sensitive as MRI in assessing hemorrhagic stroke. Hemorrhagic stroke is seen as hyperdense (bright) areas representing blood and neighboring hypodense (dark) areas representing parenchymal edema (Figure 1–13). Embolic stroke can be assessed with CT, although diffusion-weighted MRI studies (see Chapter 2 in this volume for a more detailed description of diffusion-weighted MRI) are the preferred imaging modality if ischemia or infarct is suspected. When CT is used in the acute setting (less than 48 hours after the event), ischemia or infarct appears as a hypodense (dark) intra-parenchymal lesion (Figure 1–14). Mass effect or sulcal effacement around the area of the lesions may be an associated finding. As these lesions evolve over time, they may appear isodense at approximately 1 week and then return to a hypodense (dark) appearance at approximately 3 weeks. Intravenous contrast is useful in enhancing hemorrhage or ischemia after 1–2 days. The temporal evolution of the CT appearance of ischemic strokes is presented in Table 1–5.

CT can also be useful for the detection of brain tumors. Although MRI is the preferred study for central nervous system (CNS) tumors, CT with contrast can detect larger lesions (Figure 1–15). CT with contrast is fairly sensitive for primary CNS lesions such as astrocytomas or meningiomas. On the other hand, smaller

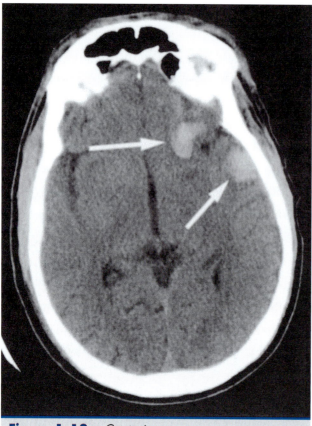

Figure 1–12.   Contusion.

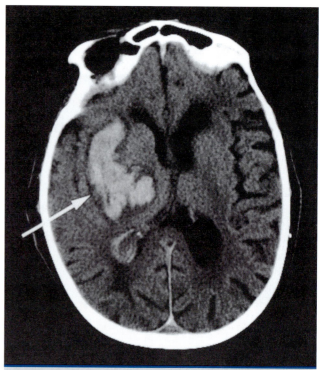

Figure 1–13.   Hemorrhagic stroke of the putamen. Bright lesion (indicated by *arrow*) represents acute bleeding; surrounding dark area represents parenchymal edema. Note mass effect of lesion on frontal horn and blood in posterior horn of the lateral ventricle.

lesions (e.g., metastatic disease) and posterior fossa tumors are more easily missed on CT. In general, solitary lesions suggest a primary CNS lesion, whereas multiple lesions suggest metastatic disease (Figure 1–16). On CT, tumors are often seen as a hypodense (dark) or isodense (gray) lesion that disturbs the normal anatomic structure of the brain. This disturbance, called *mass effect*, may be represented as displacement of anatomic structures, sulcal effacement, or midline shift. For tumors, use of contrast is helpful, because lesions will then be visible as a hyperdense (bright) area or with ring-enhancing brightness. In addition, edema is often seen as a hypodense (dark) area around the site of the tumor.

Certain types of acute infection may also produce characteristic findings on CT. By using CT with contrast, abscesses (typically from bacterial infection) may be seen as a ring-enhancing cavity within brain parenchyma (Figure 1–17). Toxoplasmosis may present as single or multiple ring-enhancing lesions (Figure 1–18). Viral infections may also be associated with certain presentations; for example, ventricular enlargement and cortical atrophy may be seen with human immunodeficiency virus (HIV) encephalopathy. Temporal lobe findings, such as edema or atrophy, may be asso-

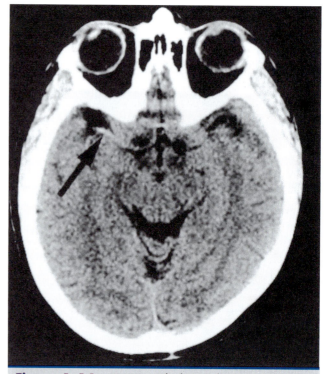

Figure 1–14.   Acute embolic stroke. Hypodense lesion is indicated by *arrow.*

Table 1–5. Temporal evolution of ischemia on CT

Setting	Time	Density	Appearance	Other
Acute	Up to several days	Hypodense	Dark	May be associated with mass effect, sulcal widening; may see decreased gray–white matter differentiation
Subacute	Up to several weeks	Isodense	Gray	Short period of hypodensity, with or without ring enhancement with contrast
Chronic	More than several weeks	Hypodense	Dark	May see volume loss with sulcal or ventricular widening

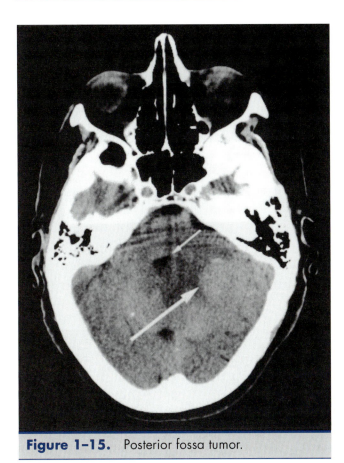

Figure 1–15. Posterior fossa tumor.

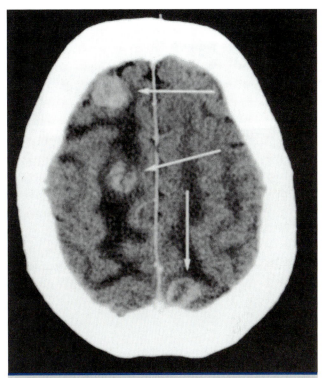

Figure 1–16. Metastatic lesions as seen on CT with contrast.

ciated with herpes simplex encephalitis (Figure 1–19).

In hydrocephalus, the production, flow, or absorption of CSF within the ventricular system is abnormal. As a result, the third ventricle and lateral ventricles often become significantly enlarged (Figure 1–20). In obstructive hydrocephalus, lateral ventricles become enlarged and may be accompanied by effacement of the sulci. Often, the space of the third or fourth ventricle may be obliterated (a compressing lesion may be seen) (Figure 1–21). Obliteration of the fourth ventricle constitutes a neurological emergency. In communicating hydrocephalus, all ventricular spaces will be enlarged (including the third and fourth ventricles). Effacement of the cortical sulci may be seen as well.

Normal-pressure hydrocephalus, which presents clinically with the classic triad of dementia, incontinence, and gait apraxia, typically resembles other types of communicating hydrocephalus. On CT, one sees dilatation of the lateral ventricles and normal or compressed sulci. Hydrocephalus ex vacuo does not arise from a problem of CSF production, flow, or absorption; rather, it arises from volume loss. While resembling the structure of other types of hydrocephalus on imaging, hydrocephalus ex vacuo is characterized by enlarged ventricles and widened sulci resulting from atrophy of brain tissue (Figure 1–22).

In severe cases of cerebral pathology, herniation of brain tissue may occur. Generally, herniation occurs when a portion of brain parenchyma becomes displaced across the tentorium cerebelli or falx cerebri.

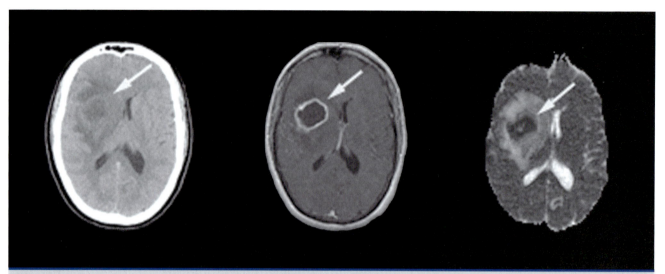

Figure 1–17. Pyogenic abscess as seen on CT with contrast, T1-weighted magnetic resonance imaging (MRI) with gadolinium contrast, and T2-weighted MRI.

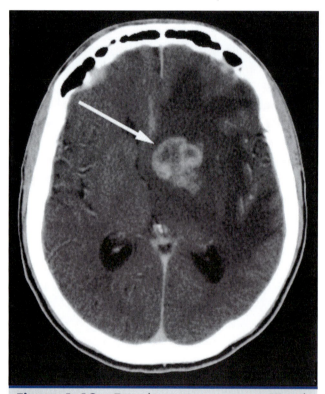

Figure 1–18. Toxoplasmosis as seen on CT with contrast.

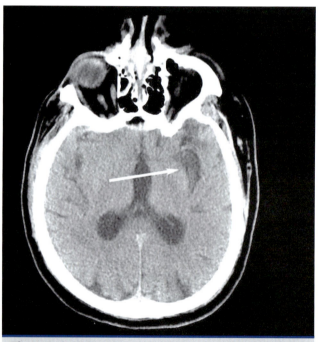

Figure 1–19. Temporal lobe atrophy consistent with herpes simplex encephalitis.

Subfalcine herniation occurs when the cingulate gyrus is displaced across the midline under the falx cerebri (Figure 1–23). Transtentorial herniation occurs when the diencephalon is displaced inferiorly across the tentorium cerebelli or the brain stem is displaced superi-

orly across the tentorium cerebelli. One type of transtentorial herniation is uncal herniation, which occurs when the uncus (the inferior aspect of the temporal lobe) is displaced across the tentorium cerebelli (Figure 1–24). Table 1–6 lists typical CT findings for common intracranial pathologies; it also indicates which study is preferred in the case of each type of suspected lesion and whether the use of contrast is recommended.

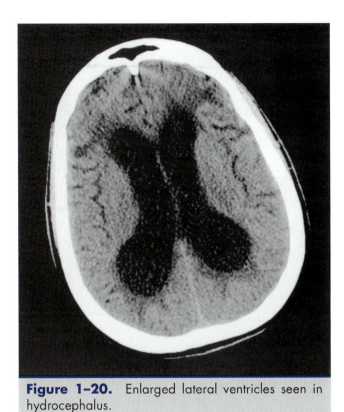

Figure 1–20. Enlarged lateral ventricles seen in hydrocephalus.

Computed Tomography–Based Research of Neuropsychiatric Disorders

After the introduction of CT, its great potential as a research tool quickly became apparent. In the 1970s, a significant amount of research using CT was aimed at uncovering the underlying structural biology of neuropsychiatric disorders. Initial CT studies of general psychiatric populations yielded little, with the majority (more than 80%) of psychiatric patients having normal CT findings. A small percentage of patients (less than 10%) demonstrated nonspecific structural abnormalities such as cerebral and cerebellar atrophy, ventricular enlargement, basal ganglia infarction, and subdural hematoma (Evans 1982; Beresford et al. 1986).

Specific psychiatric disorders were also studied with the use of CT. With the exception of studies of schizophrenia, CT studies revealed little about the structural neurobiology of psychiatric disorders. In the study of schizophrenia, however, CT played an important initial role in implicating an underlying biological substrate for the disorder. Multiple studies of schizophrenia patients demonstrated fairly consistent structural changes, with lateral ventricle enlargement

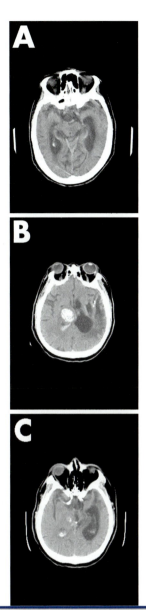

Figure 1–21. Obstructive hydrocephalus (ascending planes top to bottom [A–C]).
Note fourth ventricle evident at lower levels (**A**); obliteration of fourth ventricle around foramen of Monro (**B**) by mass lesion; and resulting hydrocephalus (**C**).

(Johnstone et al. 1976; Weinberger et al. 1979) and cerebral atrophy (Nasrallah et al. 1982) being the most reproducible findings.

Although CT-based research has never fully realized the goal of elaborating the connection between physical and mental states, it served as the foundation for a paradigm of research examining mind–body correlates through neuroimaging. Newer techniques such as MRI and functional imaging (i.e., fMRI, SPECT, PET) have taken over where CT left off and have revealed much about the biological underpinnings of neuropsy-

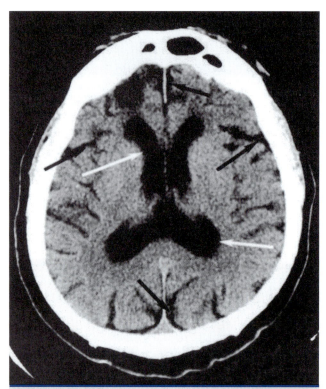

Figure 1–22. Hydrocephalus ex vacuo. *White arrows* indicate enlarged ventricles; *black arrows* indicate widened sulci.

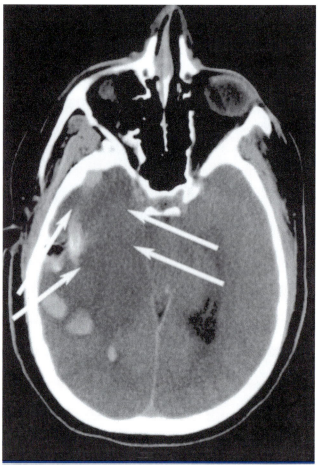

Figure 1–24. Uncal herniation. *Arrows* indicate area of downward displacement of right temporal lobe across tentorium cerebelli.

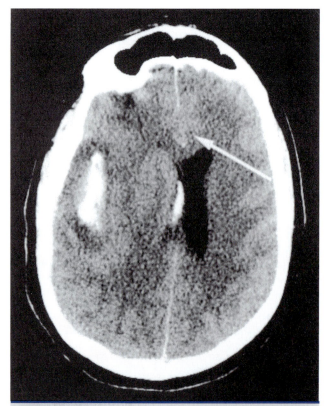

Figure 1–23. Subfalcine herniation. Right-to-left shift under falx cerebri is due to hemorrhagic process.

chiatric disease (see other chapters in this volume for further elaboration of these additional research techniques). Although CT is not the most sensitive imaging modality for identifying such underlying changes, certain psychiatric and neuropsychiatric presentations may be associated with lesions detectable on CT. Table 1–7 catalogs findings that may be visible on CT.

Clinical Indications for Neuroimaging

Neuroimaging is indicated in a variety of clinical settings, ranging from emergencies to nonacute screening situations. In the emergency setting, CT is the preferred study for evaluating abrupt change in mental status or head injury or for ruling out acute intracranial hemorrhage. In any acute clinical situation or if medical stability is tenuous, CT should be the initial imaging study used, because it takes much less time to

Table 1–6. CT findings for common pathological processes

Lesion	CT findings	Preferred study	Contrast
Subdural hematoma	Crescentic lesion between skull and brain (density varies with age of lesion)	CT	–
Epidural hematoma	Biconvex lesion between skull and brain (hyperdense)	CT	–
Subarachnoid hemorrhage	Thin lesion outlining surface of brain and CSF regions (hyperdense)	CT	–
Hemorrhagic stroke	Intraparenchymal edema (hypodense) and acute blood (hyperdense)	CT or MRI	–[a] +[b]
Embolic stroke	Hypodense intraparenchymal lesion (acute setting)	MRI	+
Tumor	Variable-density (hypo- or isodense) lesion disrupting normal anatomy; with contrast, ring-enhancing lesion	MRI	+
Contusion	Hypodense intraparenchymal lesion (acute setting)	MRI	+
Infection—bacterial abscess	Intraparenchymal cavitary lesion; with contrast, ring-enhancing lesion	CT or MRI	+
Toxoplasmosis	Multiple ring-enhancing lesions (with contrast)	CT or MRI	+
Infection—HIV with chronic CNS involvement	Ventricular enlargement, cortical atrophy, white matter hypodensities	MRI	+
Infection—herpes simplex virus	Temporal lobe edema, atrophy, uncal herniation	MRI	+
Hydrocephalus—obstructive	Lateral ventricles enlarged; third or fourth ventricles may be obliterated; effacement of sulci	CT	–
Hydrocephalus—communicating	All ventricular spaces enlarged; effacement of sulci	CT	–
Normal-pressure hydrocephalus	Dilatation of lateral ventricles; normal or effaced sulci	CT	–
Hydrocephalus ex vacuo	All ventricular spaces enlarged; widened sulci; volume loss	CT	–
Herniation—subfalcine	Cingulate gyrus displaced across the midline under falx cerebri	CT	–
Herniation—transtentorial	Diencephalon displaced inferiorly across tentorium cerebelli	CT	–
Herniation—uncal	Uncus displaced across tentorium cerebelli	CT	–

Note. +=with contrast; –=without contrast. CNS=central nervous system; CSF=cerebrospinal fluid; CT=computed tomography; HIV=human immunodeficiency virus; MRI=magnetic resonance imaging.
[a]acute; [b]subacute (>1–2 days).

obtain and is most sensitive for suspected pathologies, such as acute intracranial hemorrhage. A recent history of head trauma accompanied by loss of consciousness or a Glasgow Coma Scale (GCS) score of less than 15 warrants a CT scan. Any patient with a recent change in mental status in the presence of head trauma, age greater than 50 years, or focal neurological symptoms warrants a CT scan. In cases of cranial trauma in which fracture is suspected, time should not be spent obtaining plain-film X rays of the skull, given that CT studies (scout film and bone windows) are superior for identifying any bony lesion. MRI should not be the first study obtained, given the amount of time needed for these scans and the potential medical instability of the patient. MRI may be ordered as follow-up after CT results have been obtained and medical stability is assured. In addition, serial scanning is indicated if it is suspected that the pathological process is evolving (progressing) over time. For example, subdural hematoma, cerebral contusion, stroke, or edema

may develop over a period of hours to days. The use of serial CT (or of CT with MRI follow-up) over time is indicated if suspicion for these types of lesions is high or if the alteration in mental status does not improve (or worsens). Subsequent CT scans may be obtained at the time of acute clinical deterioration or at regular intervals (e.g., every 24–48 hours) after presentation.

CT imaging is an important diagnostic tool in the acute assessment of stroke. Although some stroke protocols employ MRI as the initial study, many protocols rely on CT as the initial study. The general rule in stroke management is to image early and often. Early use of CT can determine if the underlying disease process is hemorrhagic or embolic in nature. In addition, CT angiography (or CT myelography) may be used to assess the patency of larger vessels. Distinguishing between hemorrhagic and embolic stroke is critical, because the underlying process determines the acute management of the disease. If CT does not demon-

Table 1–7. CT findings associated with neuropsychiatric disorders

Disorder	CT findings	Studies
Schizophrenia	Volume loss of cortex, ventricular enlargement, temporal lobe volume loss	Johnstone et al. 1976; Weinberger et al. 1979
Obsessive-compulsive disorder	May be associated with structural abnormalities of caudate, white matter	Luxenberg et al. 1988
Catatonia	Has been seen with basal ganglia lesions, tumors	Gelenberg 1976
Anorexia nervosa	Has been seen with hypothalamic, third ventricle tumors	Weller and Weller 1982
Alzheimer's disease	Volume loss of cortex; ventricular enlargement, particularly medial temporal lobe	Huckman et al. 1975
Pick's disease	Volume loss of frontal, temporal lobe (lobar atrophy)	Knopman et al. 1989; Wechsler et al. 1982
Vascular dementia	Multiple small white matter lesions	Kitagawa et al. 1984
Huntington's disease	Atrophy of the caudate head	Neophytides et al. 1979
Wilson's disease	Volume loss; ventricular enlargement; hypodense lesions of putamen, pallidus	Harik and Post 1981; Ropper et al. 1979
Hallervorden-Spatz disease	Hypodense lesions in the pallidus, basal ganglia; cerebral atrophy	Boltshauser et al. 1987; Dooling et al. 1980
Wernicke-Korsakoff syndrome	Volume loss of the mammillary bodies, medial thalamus, and periaqueductal gray matter	McDowell and LeBlanc 1984; Yokote et al. 1991

strate hemorrhage and symptom onset within 3–6 hours, then thrombolytic therapy may be considered. Although the gold standard study for stroke evaluation is diffusion-weighted MRI, CT is nearly as sensitive for hemorrhage and remains a valuable tool in the management of stroke. Typically, CT will be used earlier in the course to aid in the decision-making process of acute stroke management, and diffusion-weighted MRI will be obtained in follow-up to assess ongoing progression of disease.

Neuroimaging also plays an important role in the workup and management of neuropsychiatric symptoms. An acute change in mental status may present as a change in attention, mood, personality, or cognition. Any new change in mood or personality or the development of psychotic symptoms warrants neuroimaging if the patient is older than 50 years, presents with any concurrent focal neurological signs, or has a history of significant head trauma. Neuroimaging should be a part of any workup of new-onset dementia or delirium. Once medical stability of the patient has been assured, MRI (which is more sensitive for intraparenchymal lesions) is generally preferable to CT.

Finally, neuroimaging studies are often indicated as part of the medical workup prior to an initial course of electroconvulsive therapy (ECT). Although neuro-

imaging is not currently recommended for every ECT patient, one should have a low threshold for obtaining a scan during the pre-ECT workup. Neuroimaging should be obtained if general criteria for neuroimaging are met (for any neuropsychiatric presentation) or if the patient has a history of any intracranial process, focal neurological symptoms, or psychotic/catatonic symptoms. Pre-ECT neuroimaging is useful, because it may identify an intracranial process that could potentially account for the patient's psychiatric symptoms or that could increase the risk of complications with ECT treatment. Common lesions requiring treatment or further workup prior to ECT include cerebrovascular disease, recent stroke (within several months), arteriovenous malformation, tumor, infection, or hydrocephalus. Presence of these lesions may alter the management of ECT but typically will not act as an absolute contraindication to treatment (the only absolute contraindication to ECT is critical aortic stenosis). As with any neuropsychiatric presentation, MRI is the preferred study in the pre-ECT evaluation. However, in an acute setting, if the index of suspicion for intracranial pathology is low, or if MRI is contraindicated, CT remains quite useful. Table 1–8 lists the clinical indications for neuroimaging, including which study is preferred in each case.

Table 1–8. Clinical indications for neuroimaging

Indication	Preferred study
Acute setting	CT
Medical instability	CT
Recent head trauma and one of the following:	CT
Loss of consciousness	
GCS score <15	
Acute intracranial hemorrhage suspected	CT
Stroke workup	CT or DWI (depending on protocol)
Acute change in mental status and one of following:	CT
Age >50 years	
Abnormal neurological examination results	
History of significant head trauma	
New-onset dementia	MRI or functional studies
New-onset delirium	MRI
New-onset psychosis (if age >50 years)	MRI
New-onset affective disorder (if age >50 years)	MRI
New-onset personality change (if age >50 years)	MRI
Pre-ECT workup	CT or MRI

Note. CT=computed tomography; DWI=diffusion-weighted imaging; ECT=electroconvulsive therapy; GCS=Glasgow Coma Scale; MRI=magnetic resonance imaging.

Table 1–9. Sensitivity to lesions and clinical indications for CT and magnetic resonance imaging (MRI)

CT indications and sensitivity	MRI indications and sensitivity
Emergency setting, acute trauma	Intraparenchymal lesions
Suspect acute bleed	White matter lesions
Subarachnoid hemorrhage	Ischemia/infarct
Bony lesions	Contusion
Calcified lesions	Infection
Mass effect: effacement, midline shift, herniation	Posterior fossa/brain-stem pathology
Hydrocephalus	New-onset neuropsychiatric symptoms in the subacute setting

How to Select Tests: CT and MRI

The decision of which imaging modality to order is a function of each technique's particular sensitivity for detecting a suspected pathology, its potential costs and risks, and its availability. CT and MRI are the primary neuroimaging modalities in current clinical use, with functional neuroimaging making rapid advances (particularly in the area of neuropsychiatric workup). As described in the previous section, CT and MRI each are preferable in certain situations. CT is more sensitive for characterizing certain types of pathology, such as acute intracranial hemorrhage (particularly subarachnoid hemorrhage), bony structure lesions, and calcified lesions. MRI is superior for distinguishing lesions within brain parenchyma, white matter, posterior fossa, and brain stem. Certain lesions may be equally well detected by CT or MRI; these lesions include hemorrhagic stroke, hydrocephalus, abscess (CT with contrast), and gross anatomic disruptions, such as midline shift and herniations (Table 1–9).

Additionally, each imaging modality has its own intrinsic advantages and disadvantages that the clinician needs to weigh to ensure optimal evaluation of the patient (Table 1–10). The major advantages of CT are speed, availability, and cost. The main disadvantages of CT are its relative inability to detect parenchymal lesions and the ionizing radiation load associated with each scan (though newer scanners have significantly reduced radioactive exposure). Because it involves exposure to radiation, CT is contraindicated for pregnant

Table 1–10. Comparison of CT and magnetic resonance imaging (MRI)

	CT	MRI
Speed	Rapid acquisition time: full-body scan requires less than 3 minutes	Longer acquisition time: brain scan requires approximately 10 minutes
Cost	Relatively inexpensive	More expensive
Availability	Readily available at most U.S. hospitals	Less accessible
Spatial resolution	Up to 1 mm^2	Generally superior to CT
Contraindications	Radiation load limits use in pregnant women, children	Tighter gantry and longer acquisition time increase incidence of claustrophobia Electronic devices (pacemakers, nerve stimulators) are absolutely contraindicated Metal in body a relative contraindication
Clinical	Acute setting or medically unstable patient Status postacute head trauma Suspect: acute bleed, fractures, lytic lesions, mass effect, herniation, calcified lesions	Subacute or chronic setting Superior sensitivity for acute ischemic injury Suspect: ischemia, intraparenchymal or gray–white junction, white matter lesions, contusion, infection Superior posterior fossa and brain-stem visualization

women and for children younger than 3 years. The primary contraindication to MRI is an inability on the part of a patient to tolerate the scan as a result of medical instability, claustrophobia, or agitation. Claustrophobia, experienced by approximately 5% of patients, represents a significant barrier to obtaining an MRI (although use of anxiolytic agents such as benzodiazepines may mitigate a patient's discomfort during the scan). Another important contraindication to MRI is the presence of electronic prostheses (e.g., pacemakers, neurostimulators, cochlear implants) or metal in the body (e.g., metallic objects in the eye, aneurysm clips, coils). The presence of active electronic devices represents a significant contraindication to MRI, because the magnetic field of the MRI scanner can interfere with the functioning of the device. Metal or paramagnetic objects may be caused to move within the magnetic field and are a relative contraindication to using MRI; however, recent development of MR-safe aneurysm clips or coils has essentially eliminated this contraindication in current clinical practice.

It is of great value to have a tandem of imaging modalities available for clinical evaluation, each with its individual set of sensitivities, risks, and benefits. The availability of such tools allows the clinician to select studies in an optimal fashion, taking into account a particular clinical presentation and the characteristics of a study. CT and MRI may be employed in a complementary manner. If one technique is contraindicated, the other may be an appropriate alternative. These studies may also be used in a complementary fashion; for ex-

ample, CT should be the first study ordered in an emergent situation. If additional imaging data are needed, MRI may be obtained as a follow-up study once the patient's medical stability is ensured and any rapidly progressing pathology (e.g., epidural hematoma) has been ruled out. Another example of complementary use is in the setting of new-onset neuropsychiatric symptoms. CT may be obtained if the initial presentation is acute, suspicion for organic etiology is low, or MRI is contraindicated. MRI is the preferred initial imaging study if the presentation is nonacute, the patient is medically stable, CT is contraindicated, or initial CT yields equivocal results.

References

Beresford TP, Blow FC, Hall RC, et al: CT scanning in psychiatric inpatients: clinical yield. Psychosomatics 27:105–112, 1986

Boltshauser E, Lang W, Janzer R, et al: Computed tomography in Hallervorden-Spatz disease. Neuropediatrics 18:81–83, 1987

Dooling EC, Richardson EP Jr, Davis KR: Computed tomography in Hallervorden-Spatz disease. Neurology 30:1128–1130, 1980

Evans NJR: Cranial computerized tomography in clinical psychiatry: 100 consecutive cases. Compr Psychiatry 23:445–450, 1982

Gelenberg AJ: The catatonic syndrome. Lancet 1(7973):1339–1341, 1976

Harik SI, Post MJ: Computed tomography in Wilson disease. Neurology 31:107–110, 1981

Hounsfield GN: Computerized transverse axial scanning (tomography), I: description of system. Br J Radiol 46:1016–1022, 1973

Huckman MS, Fox J, Topel J: The validity of criteria for the evaluation of cerebral atrophy by computed tomography. Radiology 116:85–92, 1975

Johnstone EC, Crow TJ, Frith CD, et al: Cerebral ventricular size and cognitive impairment in schizophrenia. Lancet 2(7992):924–926, 1976

Kitagawa Y, Meyer JS, Tachibana H, et al: CT-CBF correlations of cognitive deficits in multi-infarct dementia. Stroke 15:1000–1009, 1984

Knopman DS, Christensen KJ, Schut LJ, et al: The spectrum of imaging and neuropsychological findings in Pick's disease. Neurology 39:362–368, 1989

Luxenberg JS, Swedo SE, Flament MF, et al: Neuroanatomical abnormalities in obsessive-compulsive disorder detected with quantitative x-ray computed tomography. Am J Psychiatry 145:1089–1093, 1988

McDowell JR, LeBlanc HJ: Computed tomographic findings in Wernicke-Korsakoff syndrome. Arch Neurol 41:453–454, 1984

Nasrallah HA, Jacoby CG, MacCalley-Whitters M, et al: Cerebral ventricular enlargement in subtypes of chronic schizophrenia. Arch Gen Psychiatry 39:774–777, 1982

Neophytides AN, DiChiro G, Barron SA, et al: Computed axial tomography in Huntington's disease and persons at risk for Huntington's disease. Advances in Neurology 23:185–191, 1979

Ropper AH, Hatten HP Jr, Davis KR: Computed tomography in Wilson disease: report of 2 cases. Ann Neurol 5:102–103, 1979

Wechsler AF, Verity MA, Rosenschein S, et al: Pick's disease. A clinical, computed tomographic, and histologic study with golgi impregnation observations. Arch Neurol 39:287–290, 1982

Weinberger DR, Torrey EF, Neophytides AN, et al: Later cerebral ventricular enlargement in chronic schizophrenia. Arch Gen Psychiatry 36:735–739, 1979

Weller RA, Weller EB: Anorexia nervosa in a patients with an infiltrating tumor of the hypothalamus. Am J Psychiatry 139:824–825, 1982

Yokote K, Miyagi K, Kuzuhara S, et al: Wernicke encephalopathy: follow-up study by CT and MR. J Comput Assist Tomogr 15:835–838, 1991

Suggested Readings

Chan S, Khandji AG, Hilal SK: How to select diagnostic tests, in Merritt's Textbook of Neurology, 9th Edition. Edited by Rowland LP. Baltimore, MD, Williams & Wilkins, 1995, pp 59–106

Lewis S: Structural brain imaging in biological psychiatry. Br Med Bull 52:465–473, 1996

Novelline RA: Squire's Fundamentals of Radiology, 5th Edition. Cambridge, MA, Harvard University Press, 1997

Orrison WW Jr: Neuroimaging. Philadelphia, PA, WB Saunders, 2000

Orrison WW Jr, Sanders JA: Clinical brain imaging: computerized axial tomography and magnetic resonance imaging, in Functional Brain Imaging. Edited by Orrison WW Jr, Lewine JD, Sanders JA, et al. St. Louis, MO, CV Mosby, 1995, pp 97–144

Rauch SL, Renshaw PF: Clinical neuroimaging in psychiatry. Harv Rev Psychiatry 2:297–312, 1995

Weinberger DR: Brain disease and psychiatric illness: when should a psychiatrist order a CAT scan? Am J Psychiatry 141:1521–1527, 1984

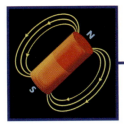

2

Magnetic Resonance Imaging

Martin A. Goldstein, M.D.
Bruce H. Price, M.D.

Technical Foundations of Nuclear Magnetic Resonance

The phenomenon of nuclear magnetic resonance (NMR) was discovered in the 1940s, setting the stage for the development of magnetic resonance imaging (MRI) for medical diagnostic use beginning in the 1970s (Taber et al. 2002). Extraordinary progress has since been made in expanding MRI's applications, producing a revolutionizing force in clinical neuroscience. Although rapidly evolving methodology continues to broaden and deepen MRI's application to research neuroscience (e.g., functional MRI), here we concentrate on the principles and utility of MRI as they pertain to clinical applications. A brief review of the technical foundations of MRI can facilitate the technology's proper use for optimal clinical advantage.

MRI exploits the magnetic properties of the atomic constituents of biological matter to construct a visual representation of tissue. The location of the NMR signal within the electromagnetic spectrum is presented in Table 2–1.

Although MRI uses electromagnetic radiation, it does not involve exposure to *ionizing* radiation, so in general patients can safely have multiple scans without concern about aggregate radiation exposure.

Table 2–1. Electromagnetic spectrum

Wave type	Wavelength (nm) (approximate)	Frequency (Hz) (approximate)
Gamma	10^{-4}	10^{20}
X ray	1	10^{18}
Ultraviolet	10^2	10^{16}
Visible	10^3	10^{15}
Microwave	10^8	10^{10}
Radio (RF), *including NMR*	10^{10}	10^5

Note. NMR = nuclear magnetic resonance; RF = radio frequency.

The degree to which a material responds to an applied magnetic field is called *magnetic susceptibility.* Whereas most body tissues have similar susceptibilities, certain atoms with unpaired electrons, which are said to be *paramagnetic* or *ferromagnetic,* have significantly greater magnetic susceptibilities.

Because the first step of MR signal generation is alignment of nuclei in an applied magnetic field, all MRI scanners have a static magnet. The strength of the static magnet affects the quality of images produced. Magnetic field strength is measured in units of tesla (T) (1.0 tesla = 10,000 gauss; for comparison, Earth's magnetic field strength is 0.00005 T, or 0.5 gauss). Scanners in current clinical use employ magnets of typically 1.5 T, although 3.0-T magnets are becoming increasingly available. Static magnets consist of circular coils surrounding a gantry onto which the patient is positioned. As an electric current is passed through the coils, a perpendicular magnetic field is generated that parallels the gantry axis. Superconductive coils, lacking significant resistance, perpetuate the electric current, with consequent production of a steady magnetic field. The coils are surrounded by liquid helium reservoirs that provide cooling to maintain superconductivity.

The balance between the number of protons and/or neutrons (collectively termed *nucleons*) in an atom determines the *angular momentum* of that atom's nucleus. If a nucleus contains either unpaired protons or unpaired neutrons (or both), the nucleus is said to have a *net spin* and consequently net angular momentum. If there are no unpaired nucleons, the nuclear angular momentum is zero. Without angular momentum, a nucleus will not *precess* when placed in a magnetic field; without precession, there can be no resonance, and therefore no NMR signal generated. Thus, only the subset of atomic nuclei having unpaired protons and/or neutrons can be used to produce a signal in NMR. Although about one-third of the almost 300 stable atomic nuclei have unpaired nucleons, and therefore have angular momentum, only a subset of these are of use for biological substrates (Lufkin 1998). Of all atoms in humans with unpaired nucleons, hydrogen (^{1}H) is the simplest, because it has only one nucleon—a proton. Hydrogen is particularly useful for medical MRI, given that hydrogen constitutes two-thirds of all atoms in the human body. In addition to its large relative chemical abundance in the human body, hydrogen is also highly magnetically susceptible, permitting high MR sensitivity (Lufkin 1998). Thus, medical MRI is essentially hydrogen NMR.

The nucleus of the hydrogen atom can be conceptualized for our purposes as essentially a proton acting as a small positively charged particle with associated *angular momentum,* or *spin.* Each proton rotates around its axis, which causes the positive charge of the proton to also spin, thereby producing a local current. This current consequently induces its own magnetic field, which then acts as a small magnet with two poles—north and south—that is, a *dipole moment* (Figure 2–1).

A vector can be used to describe the orientation and magnitude of the magnetic dipole. In the absence of any externally applied magnetic field, the vectors of the magnetic dipole moments of protons are oriented randomly in space. But because objects with a magnetic dipole tend to align when placed within an *externally applied magnetic field,* rotating protons become aligned when exposed to an MRI scanner's magnetic field (Figure 2–2).

As shown in Figure 2–2, when placed within an externally applied magnetic field, protons assume one of two possible orientations, or states: they are either parallel or anti-parallel to the applied magnetic field (Schild 1999). Protons oriented parallel to the applied field are in a lower energy state, whereas those oriented anti-parallel to the applied field are in a higher energy condition. The difference in the number of protons oriented in a parallel/low-energy state and those oriented in an anti-parallel/high-energy state is relatively small and depends on the strength of the applied magnetic field. The vector representing the large externally applied magnetic field is conventionally called B_0. The sum of all proton magnetic dipole orientations can be conceptualized as a single vector known as the *net magnetic vector,* M_0. Thus, the population of protons placed in a static magnetic field, B_0, has an M_0 whose direction is parallel to B_0 because of the slightly greater number of protons in the parallel direction (Schild 1999).

In addition to becoming aligned when placed within an externally applied magnetic field, protons, possessing angular momentum, wobble, or *precess,* around the longitudinal axis of the applied field (Figure 2–3).

Frequency of precession is known as the *resonant* or *Larmor frequency* and is proportional to the strength of the applied magnetic field, as expressed by the following equation:

$$\omega_0 = \lambda B_0$$

where ω_0 is equal to the precession frequency, B_0 is equal to the static magnetic field strength, and λ is equal to the gyromagnetic ratio, which relates static magnetic field strength to precession frequency and varies for different nuclei. Note that precession fre-

A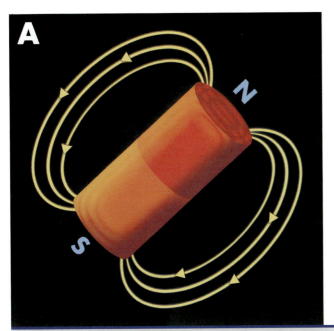

B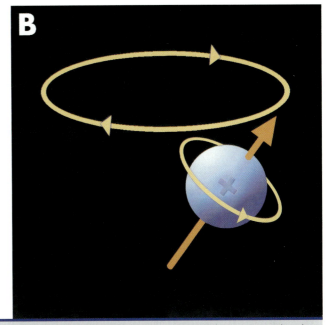

Figure 2–1. **A,** Magnetic dipole. **B,** Rotating proton with associated angular momentum and magnetic dipole.
Source. Adapted from Schild HH: *MRI Made Easy,* 5th Edition. Berlin, Germany, Schering AG/Berlex Laboratories, 1999.

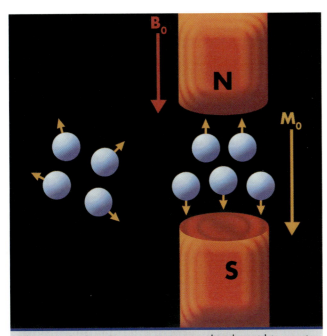

Figure 2–2. Proton magnetic dipole within static magnetic field. B_0=externally applied magnetic field; M_0=net magnetic dipole vector.
Source. Adapted from Schild HH: *MRI Made Easy,* 5th Edition. Berlin, Germany, Schering AG/Berlex Laboratories, 1999. Used with permission.

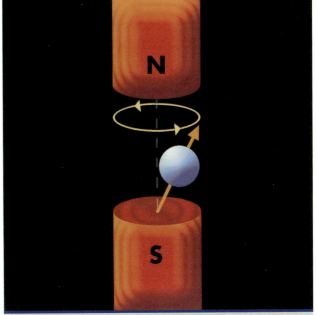

Figure 2–3. Proton precession.
Source. Adapted from Schild HH: *MRI Made Easy,* 5th Edition. Berlin, Germany, Schering AG/Berlex Laboratories, 1999. Used with permission.

quency is directly proportional to the strength of the magnetic field into which the protons are placed: the stronger the magnetic field, the faster the precession frequency. Also note that the orthogonally directed magnetic vector of each precessing proton has both longitudinal and transverse components; however, because protons are randomly precessing, the transverse components tend to cancel out, leaving only a net vertical component.

To produce an MR signal that can be detected to cre-

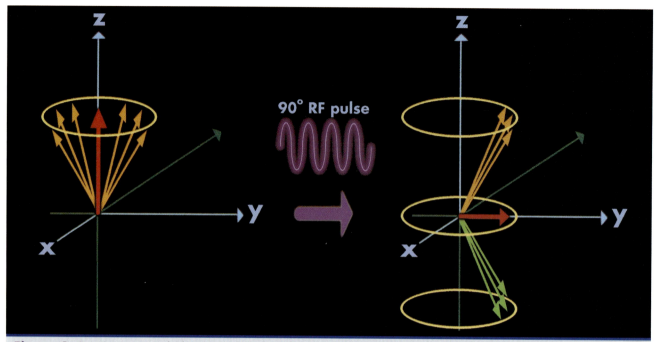

Figure 2–4. Precessional phasing. (RF=radio frequency.)

Source. Adapted from Schild HH: *MRI Made Easy,* 5th Edition. Berlin, Germany, Schering AG/Berlex Laboratories, 1999.

ate an image, the net magnetization vector must be reoriented so that a transverse component exists that can then induce a signal in a radio frequency (RF) receiver (another set of conducting coils). To move the net magnetization vector so that it acquires a transverse component, a horizontal RF pulse is applied perpendicularly to the longitudinal axis of the static magnetic field. This horizontally applied RF pulse has two effects: 1) it elevates more protons into the higher energy anti-parallel state, thereby *decreasing* the magnitude of the longitudinal component of M_0, and 2) it causes protons to precess *in phase,* thereby yielding a net transverse component of M_0 (Figure 2–4) (Schild 1999).

The applied horizontal RF pulse must be synchronized with the resonant frequency of the precessing protons in order to bring those protons into *coherence,* or *phase alignment.* Summated net precession creates a rotating magnetic vector with a transverse component alternating in time that, according to Faraday's law, can induce a current in a surrounding conducting coil, the RF receiver (Figure 2–5). This induced current oscillates at the same frequency as the transverse magnetization vector component emanating from the precessing protons. It is this electric current that is ultimately transduced into an MR image.

Only when protons are precessing in phase is it possible to detect a signal, because only the transverse com-

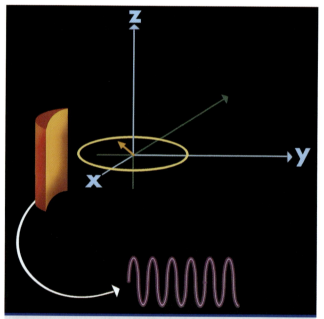

Figure 2–5. Radio frequency receiver signal induction.

Source. Adapted from Schild HH: *MRI Made Easy,* 5th Edition. Berlin, Germany, Schering AG/Berlex Laboratories, 1999. Used with permission.

ponent of the magnetization vector can be detected by RF receiver coils. The amplitude and duration of the orthogonally applied RF signal pulse can be controlled to produce variable angulation of the magnetization vec-

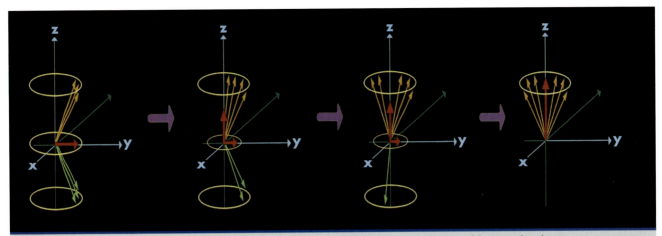

Figure 2–6. Precessional dephasing (loss of transverse vector component) and longitudinal vector recovery.
Source. Adapted from Schild HH: *MRI Made Easy,* 5th Edition. Berlin, Germany, Schering AG/Berlex Laboratories, 1999.

tor from the longitudinal toward the transverse plane.

When the horizontal RF pulse is turned off, a relaxation process occurs, with two important consequences: 1) protons that were rotating together fall out of synchrony—they *dephase,* with consequent progressive loss of the transverse magnetic vector component; and 2) protons realign with the static external magnetic field, with restoration of the longitudinal magnetic vector component (Figure 2–6).

The time required for longitudinal magnetization to recover is described by the longitudinal relaxation time constant, T1. Longitudinal relaxation is also termed *spin-lattice* relaxation, because it occurs by release of energy to the surrounding molecular lattice. This occurs more slowly than dephasing (Lufkin 1998; Schild 1999).

Dephasing occurs relatively quickly, leading to loss of the horizontal magnetization vector component and consequent progressive weakening of the detected signal. The time constant for this signal decay is *T2.* Transverse relaxation is also called *spin-spin* relaxation, because it occurs by loss of energy to adjacent spinning nuclei (Lufkin 1998; Schild 1999).

Protons dephase at different rates for two main reasons. First, because the externally applied magnetic field to which protons were originally subjected varies along a longitudinal gradient, and because precession frequency is dependent on that magnetic field strength, precession frequencies vary (i.e., absent a phasing orthogonally applied RF pulse). Second, each proton is influenced by local magnetic fields of neighboring nuclei; hence, protons in different tissues, and therefore in different magnetic environments, dephase at different rates (Lufkin 1998; Schild 1999).

The type of signal emitted as protons return to a lower energy level, progressively losing their trans-

verse magnetic vector component while regaining longitudinal magnetization, is called a free induction decay (FID) signal (Figure 2–7).

T1 is defined as the time required for 63% of the original longitudinal magnetization to be recovered. *T2* is defined as the time required for transverse magnetization to decrease to 37% of the original value. T1 typically ranges from 200 to 2000 milliseconds (msec); T2 commonly ranges from 30 to 500 msec.

Two factors affect T1: 1) the magnetic field strength (the greater B_0 is, the higher the precession frequency and the more energy that can be emitted) and 2) the composition of the surrounding lattice to which protons discharge their energy. Because the molecules composing liquids possess higher energy than the molecules composing solids, it takes longer for protons to exchange energy to the adjacent liquid milieu; hence, liquids have a *long T1* (Schild 1999). The greater the extent to which a lattice is composed of molecules that are moving more slowly, closer to the Larmor frequency at which protons precess, the more rapidly energy transfer can occur. For example, because molecular motion in fats tends to be near the Larmor frequency, spin-lattice energy transfer is easy; consequently, fats have a *short T1.*

T2 relaxation occurs when proton precessions lose phase, a process affected by inhomogeneities of the external magnetic field and of local magnetic fields within tissues. Tissues with more heterogeneous composition possess greater variations in local magnetic fields. Larger variations in these local magnetic fields cause larger differences in precession frequencies; protons consequently dephase faster, and T2 is shorter (Lufkin 1998; Schild 1999).

Because of these influences, protons have different relaxation rates and corresponding T1 and T2 time con-

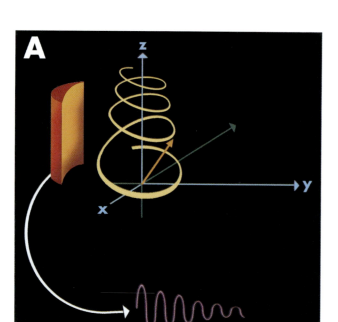
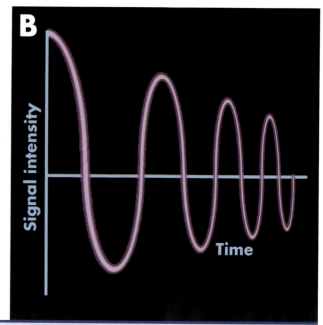

Figure 2–7. Free induction decay (FID) signal induction in radio frequency receiver.
Source.   Adapted from Schild HH: *MRI Made Easy,* 5th Edition. Berlin, Germany, Schering AG/Berlex Laboratories, 1999.

stants, depending on the molecular composition of the tissue in which they are embedded. It is these different tissue T1 and T2 time constants that provide the basis for tissue contrast in MRI. *A key strategy for how differences in T1 and T2 are exploited to generate tissue contrast involves strategic variation of timing and orientation of repetitive RF pulse delivery.* The time elapsing between pulse delivery is termed *repetition time* (TR). The characteristic knocking sound heard during image acquisition emanates from RF signal–generating coils as they repetitively deliver signal pulses.

As an example of how different tissue relaxation rates can translate into different signal intensities depending on which relaxation rate (i.e., T1 or T2) is weighted, consider Figure 2–8. The images in the figure reveal a weak cerebrospinal fluid (CSF) signal in the T1-weighted image (Figure 2–8B) and a strong CSF signal in the T2-weighted image (Figure 2–8D). The T2-weighted image also reveals white matter lesions that are not prominent in the T1-weighted image—because white matter lesions and the surrounding normal white matter have similar T1 rates (Figure 2–8A), their corresponding signals are indistinguishable. In contrast, their T2 relaxation rates are more distinct (Figure 2–8C), providing sufficient contrast in their signals to reveal the lesions.

MRI's ability to localize signals in the three-dimensional space of the brain is accomplished by using magnetic gradients—magnetic fields in which field strength changes gradually along an axis. As we have seen, precession frequency depends on ambient magnetic field strength. Therefore, protons at the same position along the magnetic gradient, corresponding to a plane perpendicular to the gradient direction, share the same precession frequency, while protons lying in other planes, experiencing different magnetic field strength, precess at correspondingly different rates. Thus, encoding of a three-dimensional volume begins by first effectively dividing the tissue mass into "slices." Then, two additional distinct orthogonally directed magnetic gradients are applied, effectively dividing each slice into rows and columns of pixels. With this encoding procedure, each pixel is imbued with a unique precessional frequency and direction. A mathematical operation called a *Fourier transformation* converts pixel data back into three-dimensional voxels, which are then assembled to form an image volume reconstruction of the original three-dimensional tissue mass. Hence, by using multiple orthogonal magnetic gradients, spatial information can be efficiently encoded. *Optimal spatial resolution currently approximates 1 cubic millimeter (partly depending on scanner strength).*

MR Image Sequence Types

Proton densities and differential T1 and T2 relaxation effects are properties intrinsic to brain tissues,

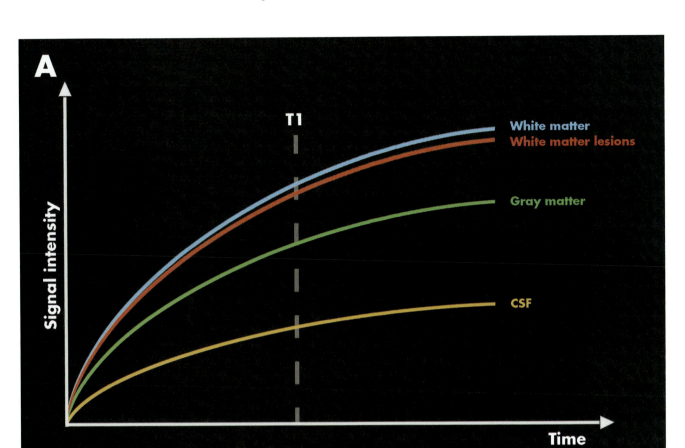

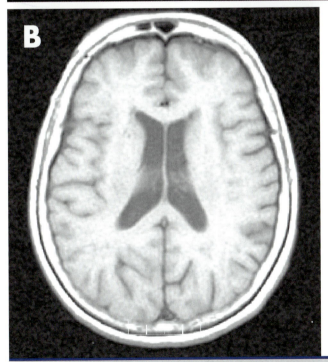

Figure 2–8. Variance in MRI signal intensity due to differential weighting of relaxation rate. **A,** T1 tissue re-laxation rates. **B,** T1-weighted axial MRI. CSF = cerebrospinal fluid.
Source. Images A and C adapted from Kandel et al. 2000.

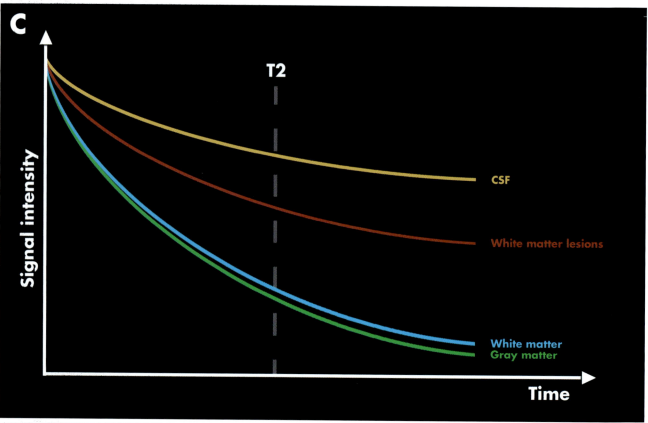

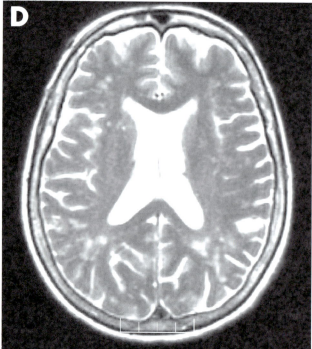

Figure 2–8 (continued). Variance in MRI signal intensity due to differential weighting of relaxation rate. **C,** T2 tissue relaxation rates. **D,** T2-weighted axial MRI. CSF = cerebrospinal fluid.
Source. Images A and C adapted from Kandel et al. 2000.

and their measurement forms the basis for the provision of differential tissue image contrast in MRI (Innis and Malison 1995). Depending on image acquisition pulse sequence selection, different tissue parameters can be differentially "weighted," thus yielding a variety of image types, each providing a unique range of diagnostic information. Because different image modalities are usually identified not by name (e.g., T1, T2) but instead by numeric values of key pulse sequence parameters set during acquisition (e.g., repetition time [TR], echo time [TE]), a brief review of some basic parameter meanings may be useful.

Note. Structural MRI orientation is according to radiological conventions; thus, images should be interpreted by considering the brain from a caudal–rostral direction, with the anterior side upward (i.e., as if viewing from the subject's feet, in the same direction as the subject is actually placed in the scanner: head first and supine). Therefore, right-sided structures are on the left side of the image, left-sided structures are on the right side of the image, anterior structures are toward the top of the image, and posterior structures are toward the bottom of the image.

T1-Weighted Images

Technical Basis

Producing a T1-weighted image involves RF stimulus delivery repetition and signal reception such that intrinsic differences in different tissues' T1 can be ex-

ploited to produce contrast. To understand this process, consider Figure 2–9.

As can be seen, two tissues, A and B, with differing T1s, have different longitudinal magnetization states at any time *before sufficient time elapses to allow the tissue with the slowest T1 to complete longitudinal relaxation*. At that point (i.e., after time 5 shown in the figure), all tissues will have fully recovered their longitudinal magnetization; hence, signal difference, and therefore tissue contrast, would be dependent primarily on proton density (Schild 1999). Thus, a *long TR* (i.e., a TR long enough to allow all tissues to complete longitudinal magnetization relaxation) does not distinguish intrinsic T1 tissue differences.

Now consider what happens if TR is *short*—that is, the second 90° pulse is delivered at a time such that different tissues, with different T1, are at different states of longitudinal magnetization recovery (Figure 2–10).

Because RF signal reception depends on the magnitude of the transverse magnetization vector component, which in turn depends on the magnitude of longitudinal magnetization at the moment of the 90° RF pulse, tissues at different longitudinal magnetization states will yield different signal intensities. As shown in Figure 2–10, use of a shorter TR *interrogates* tissues at a moment when their intrinsic T1 differences can be exploited to yield different signal intensity production, and hence tissue contrast generation. The resulting image, whose contrast is based on tissue differences in T1, is termed *T1-weighted*. A TR of less than 500 msec is considered short; a TR greater than 1,500 msec is considered long (Lufkin 1998).

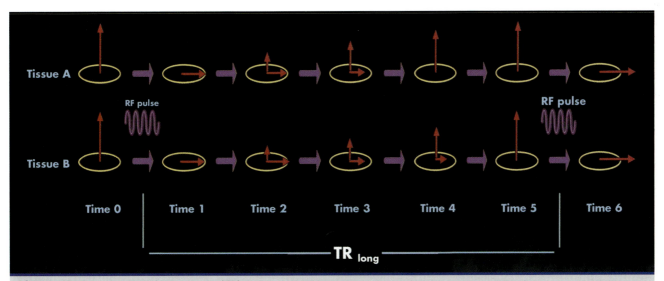

Figure 2-9. Long repetition time (TR). RF=radio frequency.
Source. Adapted from Schild HH: *MRI Made Easy,* 5th Edition. Berlin, Germany, Schering AG/Berlex Laboratories, 1999.

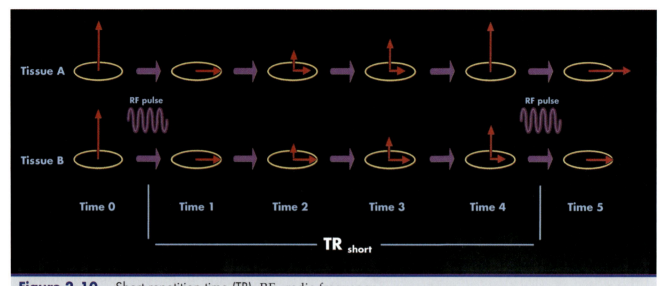

Figure 2–10. Short repetition time (TR). RF=radio frequency.
Source. Adapted from Schild HH: *MRI Made Easy,* 5th Edition. Berlin, Germany, Schering AG/Berlex Laboratories, 1999.

Use of repetitive 90° pulses to detect T1-based tissue contrast is called a *saturation recovery* sequence. An alternative method, termed *inversion recovery,* involves a pulse sequence that begins with a 180° pulse, followed by a 90° pulse, as illustrated in Figure 2–11.

The 180° pulse reverses longitudinal magnetization; all protons responsible for the net magnetic moment are inverted 180° in the applied longitudinal magnetic field. The signal received depends on the time between the 180° and the 90° interrogation pulse, which constitutes the TR for this type of pulse sequence. Just as in a saturation recovery 90°–90° sequence, an inversion recovery 180°–90° sequence will be T1-weighted if an appropriate TR is used that interrogates tissues while differences in T1 can be detected (Schild 1999).

Clinical Utility

Substances with a short T1, producing high signals on T1-weighted imaging, include fat, methemoglobin in subacute hemorrhage, and paramagnetic contrast agents. Substances with a long T1, producing low signals on T1-weighted imaging, include CSF and tissues in which any process that increases local water content has occurred (e.g., neoplasms, inflammation) (Table 2–2). *T1 images are best for visualizing normal anatomy.*

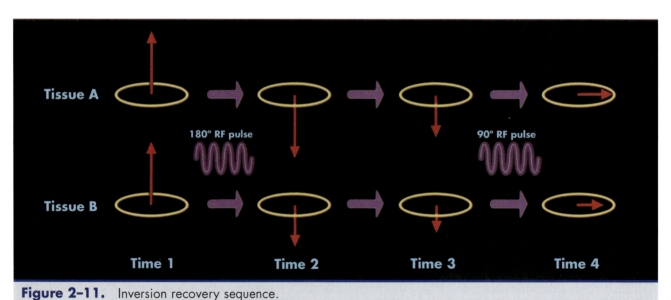

Figure 2–11. Inversion recovery sequence.
Source. Adapted from Schild HH: *MRI Made Easy,* 5th Edition. Berlin, Germany, Schering AG/Berlex Laboratories, 1999.

Table 2–2. T1 effects on appearance of T1-weighted image

Relaxation duration	Signal intensity	Tissues
Short T1	High	Fat, subacute bleeding, gadolinium
Long T1	Low	Cerebrospinal fluid, edema

Source. Adapted from Lufkin 1998.

T2-Weighted Images

Technical Basis

Generation of T2-weighted images relies on principles similar to those governing generation of T1-weighted images, although with variations in image acquisition parameter settings. Pulse sequencing is designed to interrogate tissues for the purpose of detecting intrinsic T2 differences.

A primary strategy for generating T2-weighted images involves use of a pulse sequence termed *spin-echo.* As already described, synchronous precession is ultimately undermined by magnetic field inhomogeneities of two types: 1) those arising from tissue-specific local magnetic fields of surrounding molecules and 2) those arising from applied magnetic field inhomogeneities (denoted *T2** [pronounced "T2 star"]). Both types contribute to dephasing, and spin-echo sequences are designed to try to minimize the confounding influence of T2* on the measurement of actual or tissue-specific T2 (Schild 1999).

Spin-echo pulse sequences rely on a pulse sequence strategy similar to that used in the inversion recovery method of T1-weighted imaging, except in reverse order (Lufkin 1998; Schild 1999). An initial 90° pulse generates a transverse magnetization vector component via phasing of proton precession. When the 90° pulse is terminated, dephasing soon follows, under the influence of T2 and T2*. When the 180° pulse is administered, the direction of dephasing protons is reversed. More slowly precessing protons are now ahead of faster ones. Eventually, protons with faster precession frequencies catch up, culminating in proton precession rephasing and thus detectable signal generation. This signal is referred to as an *echo* because it occurs in the absence of any stimulus delivery (Schild 1999). This process is repeated: protons again dephase, are again refocused by another 180° pulse, and so on. Thus, it is possible to obtain more than one signal by repeating the spin-echo sequence.

It is now possible to understand another key image acquisition parameter: *echo time* (TE). If we define the moment of occurrence of the echo-generated signal as the TE, it follows that the 180° RF pulse is delivered at time TE/2. If we wait another time TE/2 after delivery of the 180° spin pulse, protons rephase, at which point transverse magnetization is recovered and a signal is again generated. A long TR maximizes T2 contrast (Schild 1999).

Because applied field inhomogeneities are fixed, T2* is constant. However, because nuclei variably dephasing secondary to local inconstant inhomogeneity influences do not repeatedly catch up, and therefore do not eventually contribute to the echo-generated signal, the echo signal becomes progressively weaker. Progressive spin-echo signals therefore display decreasing intensity. Curves describing signal-intensity decrement differentially attributable to T2 and T2* effects are illustrated in Figure 2–12.

Clinical Utility

As described previously, tissues with longer T2 generate higher signals on T2-weighted images. Because the greater the fluid content of a tissue, the longer that tissue's T2 and the brighter that tissue's appearance on a T2-weighted image, T2-weighted images highlight fluid-containing regions. Thus, all normal CSF-filled spaces (e.g., sulci, ventricular system) have high signals and in the healthy brain constitute the entirety of high signal intensity. Substances with a short T2 produce low signals on T2-weighted images. Examples include iron-containing substances (Table 2–3).

Most brain lesions involve an associated change in water content. For example, brain lesions involving cellular injury (e.g., infarction) disturb cellular control of intracellular water homeostasis, causing cytotoxic edema. Extracellular inflammatory lesions (e.g., mass lesions) produce vasogenic edema. Because a final common pathway of many brain lesions involves such attendant increases in water content of brain parenchyma, T2-weighted images, which highlight tissue with higher water content, demonstrate brain pathology as higher signal intensities.

Because T2-weighted images highlight the ventricular system, they are useful for evaluating hydrocephalus. Similarly, T2-weighted images are useful for evaluating sulcal widening in cortical atrophic syndromes.

Proton Density

Technical Basis

Proton density has a direct effect on signal intensity. As previously described, only protons in hydrogen nuclei

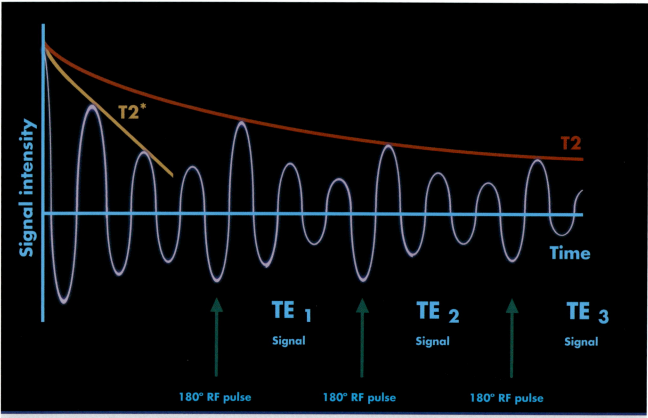

Figure 2–12. Curves describing signal-intensity decrement differentially attributable to T2 and T2* effects. RF=radio frequency; TE=echo time.
Source. Adapted from Schild HH: *MRI Made Easy,* 5th Edition. Berlin, Germany, Schering AG/Berlex Laboratories, 1999.

Table 2–3. T2 effects on appearance of T2-weighted image

Relaxation duration	Signal intensity	Tissues
Short T2	Low	Hemosiderin, deoxyhemoglobin
Long T2	High	Cerebrospinal fluid, edema, inflammation, gliosis

Source. Adapted from Lufkin 1998.

Table 2–4. Proton density (PD) effects on appearance of PD image

Proton density	Signal intensity	Tissues
Low	Low	Bone, air, calcification
High	High	Fat, fluid, edema

Source. Adapted from Lufkin 1998.

contribute to the MR signal, primarily protons of hydrogen atoms in water and fat molecules. If we set image acquisition parameters to a long TR, thereby minimizing T1-weighted signal, and a short TE, thereby minimizing T2-weighted signal, only proton density primarily contributes to signal generation.

Tissues with high proton density (PD) include fat and fluid-containing tissues. Substances with low PD include air, calcifications, and bone (Table 2–4). Because gray matter contains more water than does white matter and therefore has greater PD, *gray matter counterintuitively appears brighter than white matter on PD images* (Figure 2–13).

Clinical Utility

PD images have less clinical utility since the development of more modern image-processing strategies (e.g., gradient echo, fluid-attenuated inversion recovery); in fact, many routine image sets now do not include a PD image. Nevertheless, PD can sometimes aid interpretation of other imaging modalities by clarifying regions of pathologically low or high proton density.

Fluid-Attenuated Inversion Recovery

Technical Basis

Fluid-attenuated inversion recovery (FLAIR) is a computer-processed reconstruction of T2-weighted images that essentially involves digital suppression of high

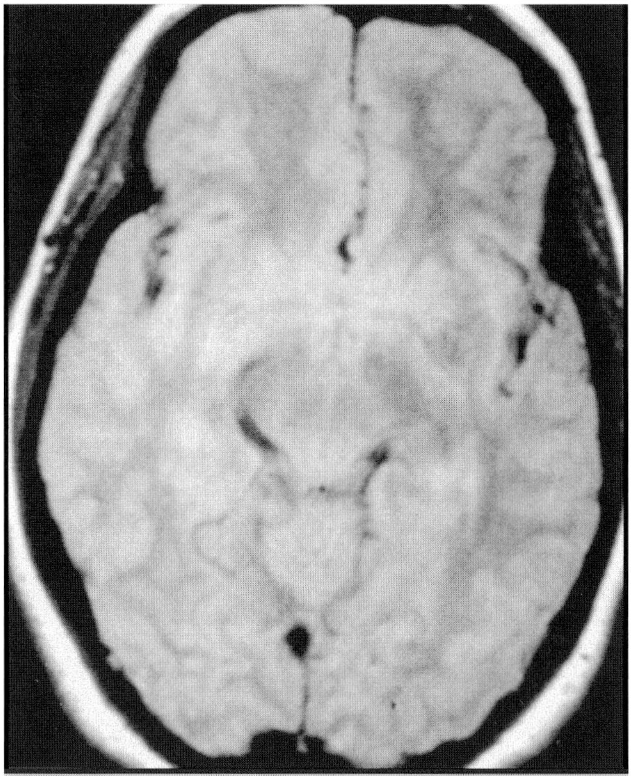

Figure 2-13. Axial proton density (PD) MRI.
Source. Reprinted from Ketonen LM, Berg MJ: *Clinical Neuroradiology (100 Maxims in Neurology*, Vol. 5). London, Oxford University Press, 1997, p. 21. Copyright 1997, Hodder Arnold. Used with permission.

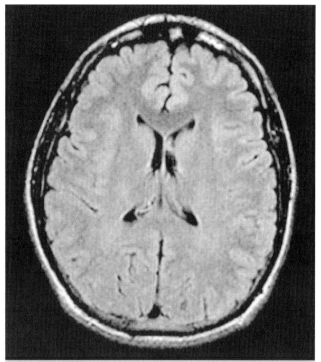

Figure 2-14. Axial fluid-attenuated inversion recovery (FLAIR) MRI.

signals emanating from *normal* fluid-filled spaces (e.g., ventricles, sulci), thereby facilitating easier visualization of increased signals emanating from any *abnormal* parenchymal water content attendant to brain lesions. Hence, FLAIR images are useful as the initial "scout" image for determining whether pathology exists and, if so, where it exists. FLAIR does not well characterize when the lesions occurred or what they are; instead, FLAIR's diagnostic power lies in providing a blueprint for use of subsequent sequences to characterize the temporal and pathological nature of the lesions.

Clinical Utility

FLAIR provides excellent contrast resolution at brain–CSF interfaces; lesions that might otherwise be obscured on routine T2-weighted images by high signals from normal adjacent CSF become conspicuous on FLAIR. Edema-generating pathology and white matter lesions, including demyelinating processes, are especially highlighted with FLAIR. This technique is therefore particularly useful in detecting small incipient demyelination lesions, thereby facilitating earlier diagnosis of related disease states (e.g., multiple scle-

rosis). Figure 2–14 presents a model FLAIR MRI.

Although subcortical white matter lesions were previously observable on T2-weighted images, FLAIR in particular has highlighted the frequency with which such lesions are discovered incidentally. Various morphological types exist; however, when found in seemingly asymptomatic individuals, these lesions often consist of multiple scattered punctate (subcentimeter) hyperintensities that are nonenhancing and are not detectable on diffusion-weighted imaging. The clinical significance of such lesions remains a target of intense clinical (e.g., neuropsychological) and pathological investigation.

Diffusion-Weighted Imaging

Technical Basis

Diffusion-weighted imaging (DWI) is a relatively new technique that detects small differences in diffusion of populations of water molecules. DWI has made its greatest impact on the diagnostic imaging evaluation of acute ischemia.

Ischemia impairs the membrane pumps that help maintain intracellular water homeostasis (intracellular hypertonicity). This results in expansion of the intracellular water compartment (cytotoxic edema), thereby producing a population of water molecules with diffusion rates different from those in extracellular space or normally functioning tissues. In clinical DWI, two scans are collected for each brain section. The first is a standard T2-weighted image. The second scan is modified during collection to make it sensitive to water molecule diffusion. Signal change differences between the first and second image are used to calculate an index of average water diffusion rate (apparent diffusion coefficient [ADC]) for each voxel. Shortly after the onset of ischemia, the ADC of ischemic brain tissue is changed secondary to cytotoxic edema. DWI detects this ischemia-associated difference in water diffusion, generating an image that, despite its extremely low resolution (see Figure 2–15), reveals even small and very recent (e.g., within an hour) ischemic regions, which are demonstrated as bright signals. Over several days, the rapid initial change in ADC is followed by a return to pseudonormal values, with dissipation of the acute ischemia-related DWI signal intensity in approximately 10 days. Hence, DWI not only detects acute ischemia but also helps to differentiate acute ischemia from chronic infarcts.

Clinical Utility

DWI has revolutionized the diagnosis of acute ischemia, including transient ischemic attacks, where DWI can reveal ischemic brain tissue even after the associated neurological deficit has normalized. DWI's sensitivity in detecting and localizing newly ischemic brain lesions enables precise differentiation of regions of acute ischemia from old infarcts, which might otherwise be difficult with conventional MR and computed tomography (CT) images. DWI's sensitivity in detecting even transient ischemia has also been employed to probe the pathophysiology of migraine headaches.

Gradient Echo

Although conventional MR images can reliably identify subacute bleeding (more than 48 hours old), acute hemorrhage is not easily detected. In addition, blood undergoes a series of appearance changes on conventional MR images (e.g., switching from dark to bright, then back to dark on T1-weighted images with time; see subsection on cerebrovascular disease, later in this chapter), which complicate interpretation (Table 2–5). Gradient echo (GE) images were developed in part to counter this significant traditional MRI weakness in revealing fresh blood and consistently detecting chronic hematoma.

GE MR images demonstrate both acute and chronic hemorrhage as extremely low signals, essentially ap-

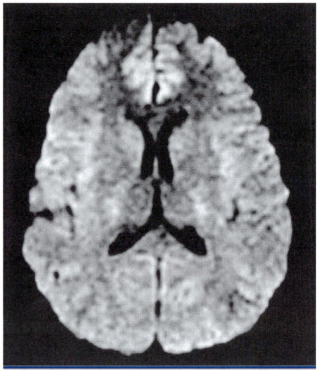

Figure 2–15. Axial diffusion-weighted imaging (DWI) MRI.

pearing black. GE can reveal any type of hemorrhage—epidural, subdural, subarachnoid, and/or intraparenchymal. Because GE can reveal a hemorrhagic component in any brain lesion, it complements the diagnostic characterizations provided by FLAIR and DWI (e.g., distinguishing hemorrhagic from ischemic strokes, demonstrating hemorrhagic conversion of large ischemic strokes). GE images can demonstrate the lobar hemorrhage of amyloid angiopathy (a common cause of intraparenchymal hemorrhage in the elderly), the hypertensive hemorrhage that usually affects subcortical structures, and the small multiple scattered punctate hemorrhages that can accompany traumatic brain injury. The latter can still be evident as dark hemosiderin deposits years later. Figure 2–16 shows a model GE MRI.

Contrast Images

Technical Basis

MR contrast agents work by altering the local magnetic environment. MR contrast materials are paramagnetic. Paramagnetic contrast agents affect image acquisition by altering the signal emanating from adjacent protons. This has the effect of enhancing both T1 and T2 relaxation efficiency (T1 predominantly) of adjacent tissues.

Table 2–5. Appearance of bleeding on MRI at various times

Stage	Time	Hemoglobin type	T1-weighted image	T2-weighted image
Hyperacute	<24 hours	Oxyhemoglobin	Dark	Bright
Acute	1–3 days	Deoxyhemoglobin	Dark	Black
Subacute				
Early	3+ days	Methemoglobin	Bright	Dark
Late	7+ days		Bright	Bright
Chronic				
Center	14+ days	Hemosiderin	Bright	Bright
Periphery	14+ days		Dark	Black

Source. Adapted from Ketonen and Berg 1997.

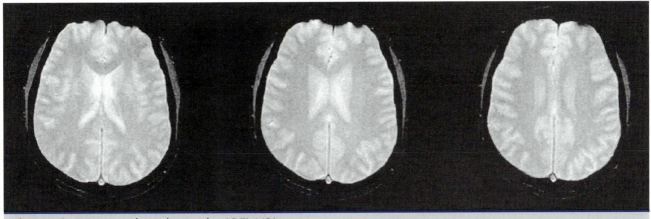

Figure 2–16. Axial gradient echo (GE) MRI.

Contrast agents most commonly used in MR are based on gadolinium. Although the free metal is toxic, gadolinium is safe for human use when chelated. The pharmacokinetics and distribution volumes of gadolinium agents are similar to those of iodinated contrast agents used for CT, and they are similarly renally excreted. However, gadolinium is much safer than iodinated radiological contrast agents, having significantly less renal toxicity (e.g., no need to prehydrate patient) and substantially less allergenic potential. Postcontrast images are usually interpreted in comparison with precontrast images. A sample postcontrast MRI is shown in Figure 2–17.

Clinical Utility

MRI contrast material is administered to aid visualization of certain lesion types. MR contrast agents diffuse from intravascular to extravascular space when the integrity of the blood–brain barrier is compromised, as occurs in many types of brain lesions. The degree and pattern of contrast enhancement provides diagnostic clues regarding the nature of the lesion. For example,

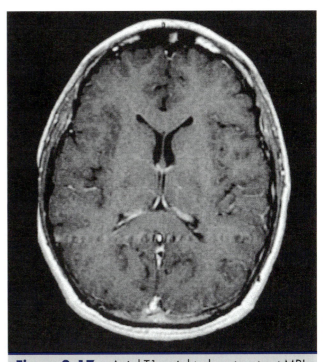

Figure 2–17. Axial T1-weighted postcontrast MRI.

whereas abscesses tend to have ring enhancement, highly vascularized tumors tend to show more solid enhancement.

Because small tumors can escape detection on noncontrast images, *gadolinium contrast is essential in evaluating patients with known or suspected neoplastic disease* (primary or metastatic masses, leptomeningeal disease). Most tumors at least partially enhance; both blood–brain barrier dysfunction and vascular proliferation are responsible for the enhancement. For most tumors, the degree of tumor enhancement tends to correlate with degree of malignancy.

Contrast images are essential for the neuroimaging evaluation of a new seizure disorder, because certain lesions acting as epileptogenic foci may be visualized only after contrast administration.

Demyelinating lesions associated with multiple sclerosis tend to enhance when acute. Hence, although demyelination in general is best demonstrated on FLAIR, contrast images can help differentiate acute from chronic pathology.

In theory, any type of image weighting can be paired with MR contrast administration. However, because T1-weighted images offer the best means of structural resolution (and T1 is more affected by contrast effects), T1-weighted images are the usual image type for which pre- and postcontrast images are generated.

Diffusion Tensor Imaging

Technical Basis

Diffusion tensor imaging (DTI) is a powerful new imaging technique that provides a means of evaluating brain structure, particularly white matter integrity, at a microstructural level. A basic understanding of the principles of DTI can help the clinician appreciate its clinical applications.

DTI exploits water's differential diffusion along (parallel to) versus across (perpendicular to) axons. This property of water provides a mechanism for assaying axonal direction and integrity. (Although DWI also relies on changes in water diffusion to detect acute ischemia, DWI provides only limited information about the *direction* of water diffusion.)

In DTI, a minimum of seven images is acquired for each brain slice (Taber et al. 2002). As in DWI, one image is simply a standard T2-weighted image. The rest of the images are modified during collection to make them sensitive to water movement in different directions (Taber et al. 2002). From the complete set of seven images, a matrix describing diffusional speed in each

direction is calculated for every image voxel. This matrix of diffusion vectors is the diffusion *tensor* and gives the technique its name (Taber et al. 2002).

Normally, water molecule diffusion is similar in all directions; such diffusion is termed *isotropic* (Figure 2–18A). Water diffusion in gray matter is relatively isotropic. In white matter, however, diffusion occurs significantly more rapidly parallel to versus across axons. Consequently, water diffusion in white matter is more directional, a property termed *anisotropic* diffusion (Figure 2–18B).

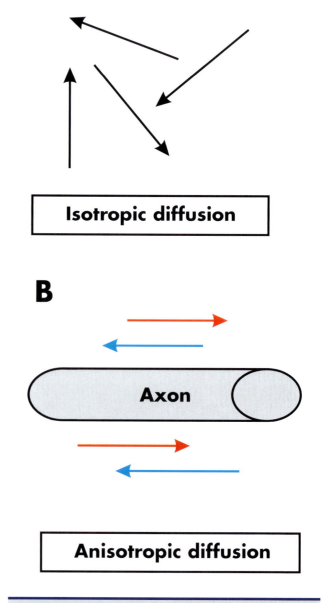

Figure 2–18. Isotropic **(A)** and anisotropic **(B)** water molecule diffusion.

Because anisotropy is determined by white matter tracts, the degree of anisotropy within each voxel can provide an index for white matter structural integrity. DTI can thereby help identify pathological sites. The direction of anisotropy can provide further information about fiber direction that can be used for mapping fiber tracts, which may be altered by developmental abnormalities, degenerative disease, or acquired pathology (Taber et al. 2002).

One way of displaying fiber tract directionality is by using directionally coded color (Taber et al. 2002). The principal direction of diffusion in each voxel is represented by a color scheme in which a set color is assigned to each major direction (anterior–posterior, left–right, supero–inferior) (Taber et al. 2002) (Figure 2–19).

Although promising, DTI is a relatively new modality and requires significant refinement. The ultrafast echo-planar MR scanning method used for DTI acquisition is vulnerable to artifacts in areas of magnetic field inhomogeneity, such as brain–bone and brain–air interfaces (Taber et al. 2002). DTI requires the combining of information from many images and therefore is sensitive to patient movement. Because voxels are large relative to some of the white matter structures examined, images can be particularly vulnerable to partial volume artifacts (Taber et al. 2002). The technique is also especially susceptible to errors at points where fibers cross or acutely converge ("kiss") or diverge.

Clinical Utility

Although DTI currently remains primarily a research tool, clinical applications are being developed. Indeed, DTI offers great promise for the evaluation of a variety of neuropsychiatric disease states. Here we briefly review examples of specific neurodevelopmental, neurodegenerative, traumatic, and primary psychiatric disease states in which DTI has revealed abnormalities that were undetected on conventional MRI.

An example of DTI's application in developmental disorders is Klingberg et al.'s (2000) report of left temporoparietal region anisotropy decrease correlating with reading impairment in adults diagnosed with developmental dyslexia.

DTI studies of patients with schizophrenia have found decreased frontal white matter anisotropy, suggesting axonal abnormalities (Taber et al. 2002). Another study found decreased anisotropy diffusely spread across prefrontal, temporoparietal, and parietal-occipital regions (Lim et al. 1999). DTI examinations of the corpus callosum in patients with schizophrenia

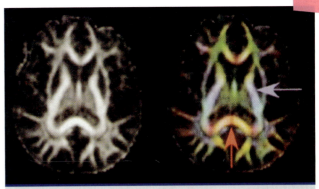

Figure 2–19. Diffusion tensor imaging (DTI). Anisotropy map *(left)* and color-coded DTI *(right)* of a healthy control subject.
Source. Reprinted from Taber KH, Pierpaoli C, Rose SE, et al.: "The Future for Diffusion Tensor Imaging in Neuropsychiatry." *Journal of Neuropsychiatry and Clinical Neurosciences* 14:1–5, 2002. Copyright 2002, American Psychiatric Publishing, Inc. Used with permission.

have also found reduced anisotropy (Foong et al. 2000).

Acquired brain injury has become an especially prominent domain of DTI application. An example of DTI's application in traumatic brain injury (TBI), as reported by Rugg-Gunn et al. (2001), is shown in Figure 2–20. Although standard T1-weighted and T2-weighted images were normal in this patient following motor vehicle accident-related TBI, DTI revealed abnormalities functionally neuroanatomically consistent with clinical signs that included left-sided motor deficit (right internal capsule), as well as executive dysfunction and personality change (right frontal subcortical). In a contrasting example suggesting the utility of DTI for demonstrating functional preservation of tissue appearing acutely or subacutely abnormal on conventional MRI, Werring et al. (1998) reported a case of TBI in which later motor recovery correlated with preserved motor pathway anisotropy.

DTI has also been used to investigate neurodegenerative disorders. For example, Rose et al. (2000) used DTI to study patients who had been given a diagnosis of probable Alzheimer's disease (AD). When compared with age-matched control subjects, patients with probable AD demonstrated reduced anisotropy in the splenium of the corpus callosum, superior longitudinal fasciculus, and left cingulate. Changes in anisotropy of the splenium correlated well with Mini-Mental State Examination scores (Rose et al. 2000).

As these reports suggest, DTI has broad potential neuropsychiatric applications for in vivo demonstration of subtle microstructural pathology previously undetected by conventional neuroimaging modalities.

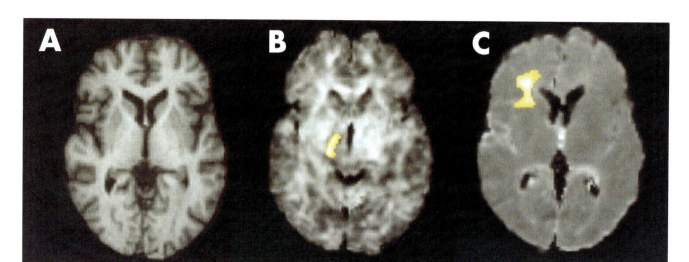

Figure 2–20. T1 and DTI MRIs of a patient with traumatic brain injury.
A, Normal T1 image. **B,** DTI MRI revealing an area of significantly reduced anisotropy is demonstrated in the posterior limb of the right internal capsule *(yellow),* concordant with the patient's motor signs. **C,** DTI MRI revealing an area of reduced anisotropy in the right frontal white matter *(yellow),* concordant with the patient's neuropsychological findings (executive deficits).
Source. Reprinted from Taber KH, Pierpaoli C, Rose SE, et al.: "The Future for Diffusion Tensor Imaging in Neuropsychiatry." *Journal of Neuropsychiatry and Clinical Neurosciences* 14:1–5, 2002. Copyright 2002, American Psychiatric Publishing, Inc. Used with permission.

Image Anatomic Slice Orientation

One of the great advantages of MRI is its capacity to produce multiplanar images. Whereas CT is limited to axial orientation, MR can image in any plane. Because magnetic gradients can be produced in multiple directions, axial, coronal, and sagittal images can be generated without changing the patient's orientation.

Axial Slices

Axial images are the best slice orientations with which to begin MRI assessment, because they provide important basic information regarding overall parenchymal and CSF space structural integrity. Initial axial image sequences routinely include T1, T2, FLAIR, DWI, and GE.

Axial T1

Gross hemispheric abnormalities (e.g., mass effects), basal ganglia size and symmetry, ventricular system size and symmetry, cortical gyri and sulci deformations, and convexity abnormalities can be quickly and easily evaluated. T1 axial images are essential in surveying for convexity abnormalities (e.g., subdural hematoma). T1 axial images provide surrounding structural information (thereby complementing T2 images) for the initial evaluation of the ventricular system. Parenchyma bordering the lateral ventricle frontal horns, temporal horns, posterior horns, third ventricle, and fourth ventricle can be assessed in turn on serial slices. In determining hydrocephalus, assessment of ventricular dilatation out of proportion to peripheral cerebral atrophy can in part be evaluated by assessing lateral ventricular temporal horn widths and superior slice sulci depths. Figure 2–21 shows a model T1-weighted axial MRI.

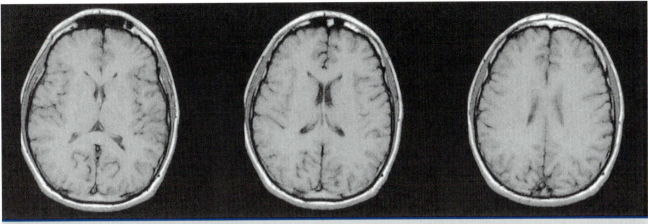

Figure 2–21. Axial T1-weighted MRI.

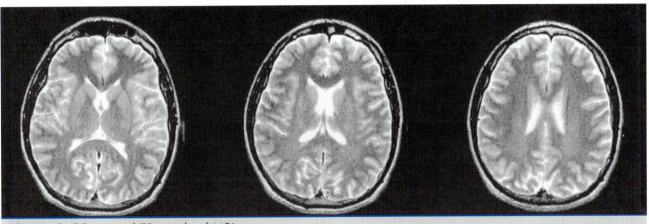

Figure 2–22. Axial T2-weighted MRI.

Axial T2

T2 axial images are used to evaluate all CSF spaces, including basal cisterns, ventricles, and sulci. T2 signal hyperintensities associated with parenchymal pathology are usually evident but can be obscured by normal CSF T2 signal, especially subjacent to ventricular spaces and sulci. Figure 2–22 shows a model T2-weighted axial MRI.

Axial FLAIR

Axial FLAIR images have become the key initial survey images used in evaluating for the presence of brain pathology, providing the blueprint for determining the existence and location of brain pathology for which subsequent sequences are used to characterize temporal and pathological attributes. Figure 2–23 shows a model axial FLAIR MRI.

Axial DWI

Axial DWIs are typically the only DWI images routinely obtained. They are used to evaluate for acute ischemia (Figure 2–24).

Axial GE

Axial GEs are typically the only GE images routinely obtained. They are used to evaluate for the presence of acute hemorrhage, chronic hematoma, and residua of old bleeding (Figure 2–25).

Axial T1 With Gadolinium Contrast

Axial slices are the typical orientation in which post-gadolinium T1 images are obtained (Figure 2–26).

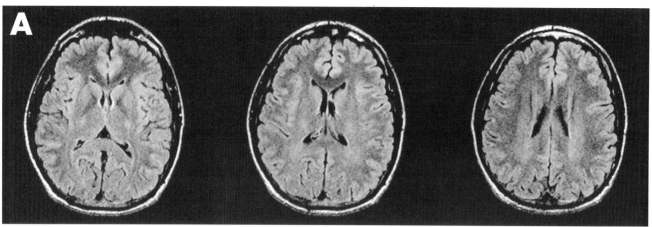

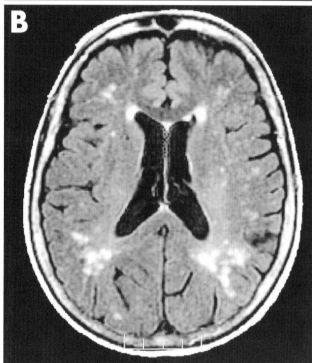

Figure 2–23.   Axial fluid-attenuated inversion recovery (FLAIR) MRI showing **(A)** normal findings and **(B)** FLAIR-evident lesions.

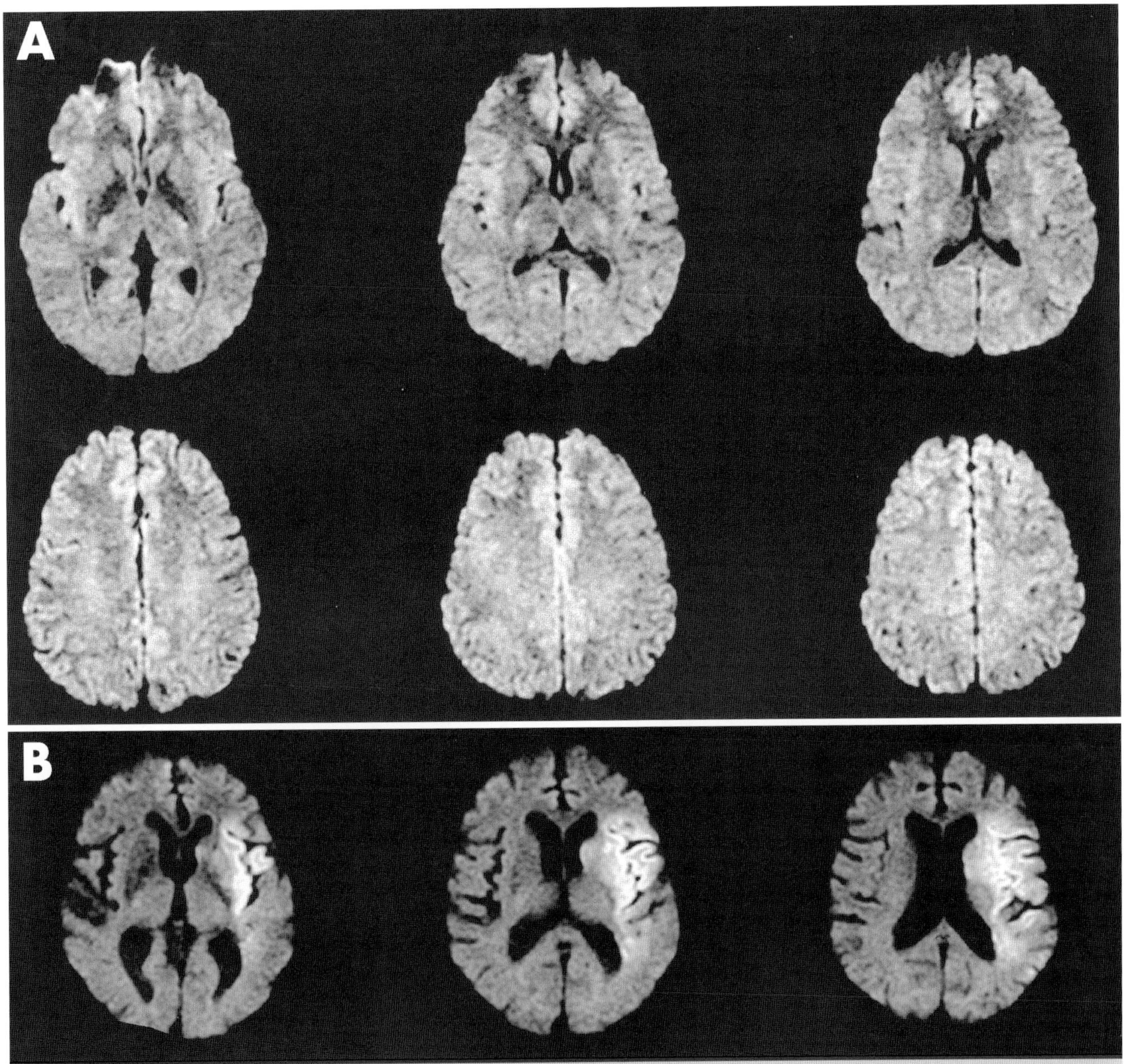

Figure 2-24. Axial diffusion-weighted imaging (DWI) MRI showing **(A)** normal findings and **(B)** acute or subacute stroke.

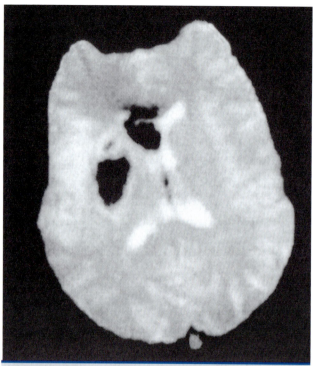

Figure 2–25. Axial gradient echo (GE) MRI showing hemorrhage.
Source. Reprinted from Nighoghossian N, Hermier M, Adeleine P, et al.: "Old Microbleeds Are a Potential Risk Factor for Cerebral Bleeding After Ischemic Stroke: A Gradient-Echo T2*-Weighted Brain MRI Study." *Stroke* 33:735–742, 2002. Copyright 2002, Lippincott Williams & Wilkins (www.lww. com). Used with permission.

Coronal Slices

Coronal slice orientation images are especially relevant for evaluating psychiatric symptoms, given that inferomedial structures—including the amygdala, the hippocampus, and other limbic and paralimbic regions (which increasingly are being recognized as key substrates of the neurocircuitry underlying affective and cognitive disturbance)—have an anterior–posterior longitudinal orientation that is best assayed with coronal slicing. Coronal images are also useful in evaluating normal structures that cross the midline (i.e., corpus callosum) and in assessing pathology for midline crossing (e.g., malignant brain tumors such as glioblastoma multiforma). Coronal slices tend not to be performed as part of a routine MRI protocol; it is therefore often necessary to specifically request them.

Coronal T1

Coronal T1 images are best for evaluating anatomy of the anterior–posterior oriented structures described above (e.g., assessing for hippocampal atrophy or asymmetry) (Figure 2–27).

Coronal FLAIR

Coronal FLAIR images are especially useful for evaluating pathology in inferomedial temporal structures (e.g., detection of seizure foci for temporal lobe epilepsy, such as mesiotemporal sclerosis) (Figure 2–28).

Coronal T1 With Gadolinium Contrast

Coronal T1 images with gadolinium contrast can be requested as follow-up images to facilitate evaluation of mediolateral extent of lesions demonstrating enhancement on initial axial T1 postgadolinium images.

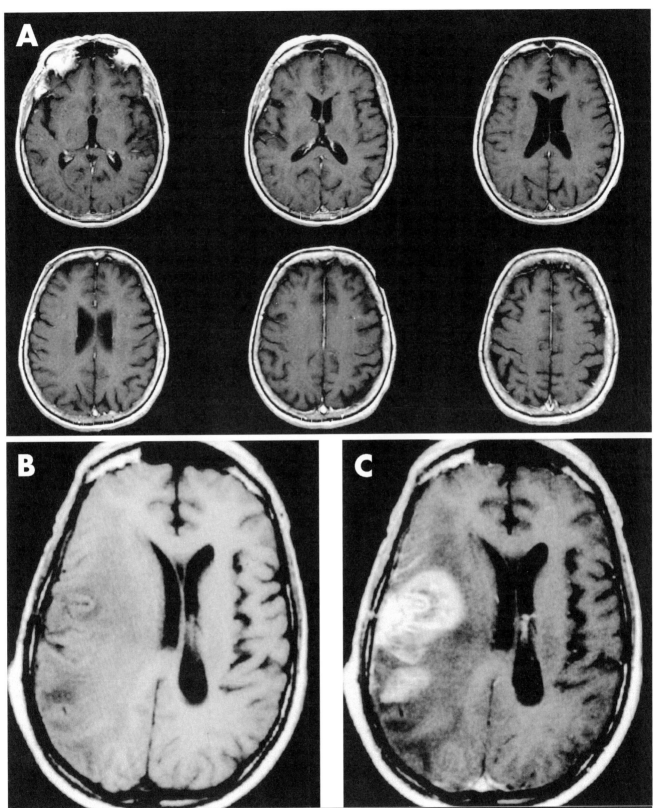

Figure 2–26. Axial T1-weighted MRI with gadolinium contrast.
A, Postcontrast T1-weighted axial MRI showing normal findings. **B,** Precontrast T1-weighted axial MRI showing mass effects. **C,** Postcontrast T1-weighted axial MRI showing contrast-enhancing mass lesion.
Source. Images B and C reprinted from Fink KL, Rushing EJ, Schold SC: "Neuro-Oncology," in *Atlas of Clinical Neurology.* Edited by Rosenberg RN. Philadelphia, PA, Butterworth-Heinemann, 1998, p. 8.11. Copyright 1998, Current Medicine, Inc. Used with permission.

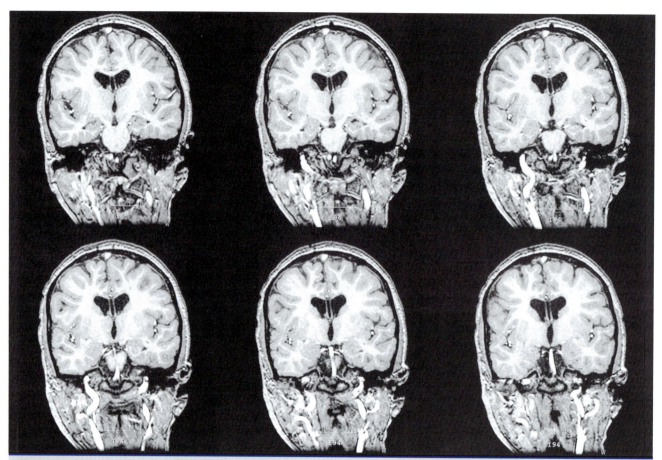

Figure 2–27. Coronal T1-weighted MRI.

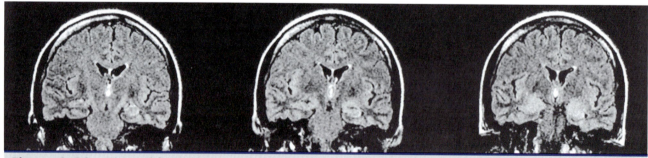

Figure 2–28. Coronal fluid-attenuated inversion recovery (FLAIR) MRI.

Sagittal Slices

Sagittal images are useful for lobar comparisons, visualizing midline anterior–posterior oriented structures (e.g., corpus callosum) and midline rostrocaudal structures (e.g., Sylvian aqueduct), as well as evaluating the rostrocaudal positioning of the neuraxis. T1-weighted sequences are typically the only sagittal images produced in routine protocols.

Sagittal T1

Sagittal T1 images are especially helpful for evaluating selective lobar atrophy syndromes (e.g., frontotemporal dementias such as Pick's disease). Corpus callosal abnormalities (e.g., dystrophic and atrophic syndromes, bowing secondary to communicating hydrocephalus) can also be demonstrated. Midline ventricular system structures (e.g., Sylvian aqueduct) can best be evaluated by medial sagittal slicing to ensure complete patency of the ventricular system. Sagittal T1 images are helpful for evaluating downward displacement of the neuraxis associated with neurodevelopmental abnormalities (e.g., Arnold-Chiari malformation) and acquired disease (e.g., intracranial hypotension). Figure 2–29 shows a sample T1-weighted sagittal MRI.

Sagittal FLAIR

Sagittal FLAIR images are especially useful for determining the pattern of white matter lesions detected on axial FLAIR images. Figure 2–30 shows a model sagittal FLAIR MRI.

Sagittal T1 With Gadolinium Contrast

Sagittal T1 images with gadolinium contrast should be ordered only as follow-up for detailed evaluation of the anterior–posterior and supero–inferior extent of enhancing lesions discovered on postcontrast axial T1 images.

Pituitary Protocol

Given the importance of the hypothalamic-pituitary-adrenal cortical axis to neuropsychiatric function, imaging the pituitary is sometimes useful, especially in the context of ancillary end-organ evidence of possible pituitary dysfunction (e.g., thyroid abnormalities). A pituitary protocol essentially comprises thin coronal, sometimes supplemented by sagittal, slices through the pituitary. Primary pituitary abnormalities (e.g., cysts, neoplastic lesions) can be well demonstrated. Potential pathology involving surrounding structures can also be visualized (e.g., sella turcica abnormalities, including sellar masses and empty sella syndrome, both with potential implications for pituitary function).

Magnetic Resonance Angiography

Imaging the cerebrovasculature is rarely indicated for diagnostic evaluation of primary psychiatric disorders. However, a variety of cerebrovascular disease states (e.g., arteriovenous malformations) can have associated psychiatric symptoms—for example, by means of mass effect, perfusion defects, and/or functioning as epileptogenic foci. Magnetic resonance angiography (MRA) has revolutionized visualization of cerebrovasculature by providing a noninvasive means of imaging large and medium-sized intracranial blood vessels. A complementary technique, magnetic resonance venography (MRV), images dural venous sinuses and other components of the intracranial venous system. Neck MRAs have become extremely useful for noninvasive imaging of carotid arteries. Sample MRA and MRV images are presented in Figure 2–31.

Model Image Sequence Interpretation Paradigm: How to Read an MRI

Although final interpretations of MRIs should be left to physicians trained in neuroradiology, being able to read one's own patients' MRIs can be diagnostically powerful in that it can facilitate a synergistic linkage of clinical and neuroimaging data. The key is arranging images in a sequence that allows relevant data from the images to be logically extracted and synthesized into a meaningful clinical interpretation. A paradigm for this process is shown in Figure 2–32.

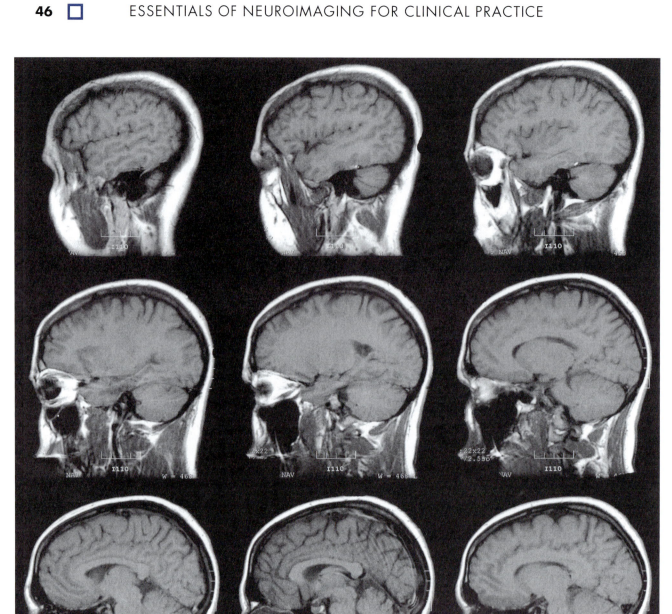

Figure 2–29. Sagittal T1-weighted MRI.

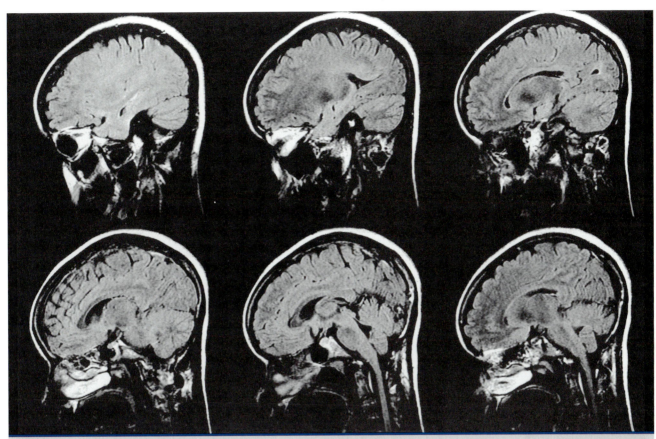

Figure 2–30. Sagittal fluid-attenuated inversion recovery (FLAIR) MRI.

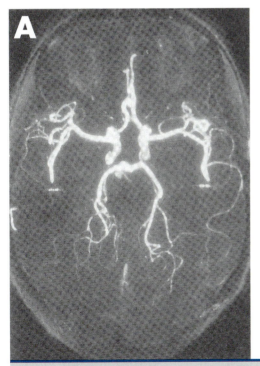

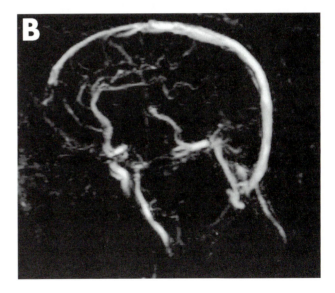

Figure 2–31. Magnetic resonance angiography **(A)** and venography **(B)**.

Source. Image A reprinted from Aygün N, Masaryk TJ: "MR Angiography: Techniques and Clinical Applications," in *Magnetic Resonance Imaging of the Brain and Spine.* Edited by Atlas SW. Philadelphia, PA, Lippincott Williams & Wilkins, 2002, p. 992. Copyright 2002. Used with permission.

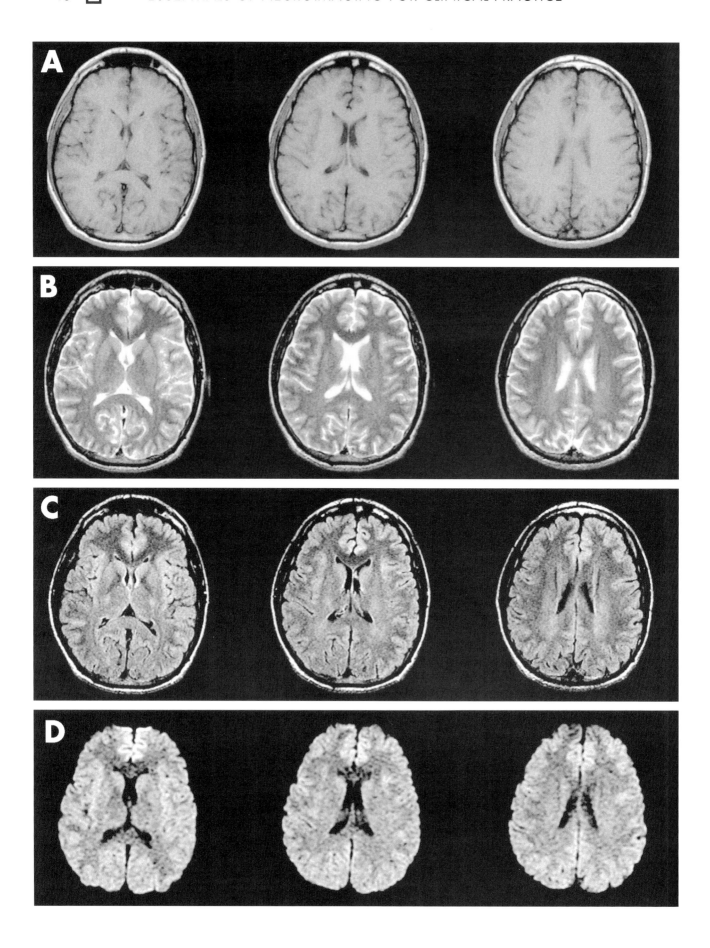

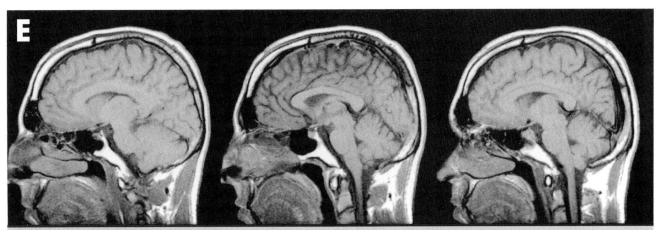

Figure 2–32. Model image sequence interpretation paradigm.
A, Axial T1-weighted MRI. **B,** Axial T2-weighted MRI. **C,** Axial FLAIR MRI. **D,** Axial DWI MRI. **E,** Sagittal T1-weighted MRI.

Review of Empirical Findings on Structural Neuroimaging Relevant to Clinical Psychiatry

Almost any intracranial abnormality can potentially produce psychiatric clinical manifestations (Bertelson and Price 2003). Table 2–6 summarizes some of the major categories of MRI-detectable pathologies with potential relevance to clinical psychiatry.

Given the existence of seemingly countless etiologies with potential for protean disturbances of affect, cognition, perception, and/or behavior, the clinical challenge is to determine when a neuroimaging study is indicated and what specific imaging modalities should be employed to optimize diagnostic sensitivity and specificity. More prospective controlled studies are needed to determine the diagnostic yield of MRI across a range of patient populations and disease states, as well as the impact of MRI on treatment decisions and outcome (Rauch and Renshaw 1995). Only then can optimal guidelines be developed to inform clinicians. For now, we review a sample of MRI findings potentially associated with psychiatric phenomena to reinforce MRI principles and to further highlight MRI's potential utility in clinical psychiatry.

General Psychiatric Populations

There have been multiple attempts to determine the association between abnormal structural MRI scan findings and primary psychiatric disease. Initial studies suggested that almost 20% of patients with a primary psychiatric disorder had evidence of a focal abnormality on brain MRI (Rauch and Renshaw 1995). Many of these studies, however, were methodologically compromised (Rauch and Renshaw 1995).

One of the more ambitious efforts to characterize MRI abnormalities in psychiatric patient populations was conducted by Rauch and Renshaw (1995). Over a 5-year period at McLean Hospital, 6,200 inpatients—consisting of consecutive referrals for MRI (representing approximately 40% of all admissions to the hospital over the same period)—underwent brain MRI. Table 2–7 summarizes prevalences of unanticipated findings, some with potential management implications.

The overall yield of unexpected, remediable pathology was low (Rauch and Renshaw 1995). The most common findings were hemorrhage and white matter abnormalities. Ninety-nine patients, or 1.6%, were noted to have findings that might lead to a change in clinical management. The authors inferred from the prevalence of MRI white matter abnormalities that the most common undetected diagnosis was multiple sclerosis (although multiple sclerosis cannot be diagnosed solely on the basis of MRI findings).

Other early studies, driven by MRI's power for revealing white matter disease relative to CT, also found increased prevalence of white matter lesions in psychiatric populations. When subsequent studies revealed that many healthy control subjects have white matter abnormalities of no apparent clinical significance, investigators and clinicians began to question the relevance of white matter lesions in psychiatric illness. Nevertheless, some evidence suggests that white matter lesions are indeed more prevalent in certain psychi-

Table 2–6. Examples of MRI-detectable brain pathology that can manifest clinically as psychiatric disturbance

Pathological class	Syndrome	MRI modality	Example finding

Ventricular system/CSF volume abnormalities	Hydrocephalus
	    Ex vacuo (e.g., atrophy)
	    Communicating (e.g., NPH)
	    Obstructive
		Axial T1, T2; sagittal T1	Variable ventricular dilatation

Cerebrovascular	Hemorrhagic		
	Epidural	GE	Expanding subcranial hypointensity
	Subdural	GE, T2, FLAIR	Convexity abnormality
	Subarachnoid	GE	Subarachnoid hypointensities
	Intraparenchymal	GE	Variable hypointensities
	Ischemic		
	Small-vessel lacunar	Acute: DWI, FLAIR	Focal punctate subcortical hyperintensity
		Chronic: FLAIR	Scattered small subcortical hyperintensities
	Large-vessel thromboembolic	Acute: DWI, FLAIR	Large focal cortical hyperintensity
		Chronic: FLAIR	Large focal cortical hyperintensity
		Old: T1	Focal encephalomalacia, atrophy
	Aneurysm	MRA	Vascular abnormality
	Arteriovenous malformation	MRA	Vascular abnormality
	Dural venous thrombosis	MRV	Flow deficit
Metabolic	Wilson's disease	Coronal T1, FLAIR	Cystic putamenal lesions
	Mitochondrial encephalopathy lactic acidosis and stroke (MELAS)	FLAIR	Variable infarcts
Inflammatory	White matter (e.g., multiple sclerosis)	Sagittal FLAIR	Dawson's fingers (in multiple sclerosis)
	Vasculature (e.g., vasculitis)	FLAIR, MRA	Focal punctate lesions
	Idiopathic (e.g., sarcoidosis)	T1, T1 + gad	Variable enhancement
Neoplastic	Tumor		
	Primary	T1, T1 + gad, FLAIR	Variably enhancing mass lesions
	Metastatic	T1, T1 + gad, FLAIR	Variably enhancing mass lesions
	Leptomeningeal disease	T1, T1 + gad, FLAIR	Leptomeningeal enhancement
Infectious	Encephalitis	T1, T1 + gad, FLAIR	Variable enhancement, edema
	Meningitis	T1, T1 + gad	Edema, enhancement
	Abscess	T1, T1 + gad	Ring-enhancing mass
Toxic	Alcohol	Axial T1	Cerebellar vermis atrophy
	Heavy metal	Coronal T1, T2, FLAIR	Basal ganglia abnormalities
Trauma	Acute	T1, DWI, GE, FLAIR	Acute hemorrhage, edema
	Chronic	T1, GE, FLAIR	Petechial hemosiderin deposits, encephalomalacia
Neurodegenerative	Alzheimer's disease	Coronal T1	Hippocampal atrophy ± temporal/parietal/generalized atrophy
	Dementia with Lewy bodies	Axial, coronal T1	Similar to Alzheimer's disease
	Frontotemporal dementia	Sagittal T1	Frontal and/or temporal gyral knife-edge atrophy
	Huntington's disease	Coronal T1	Bilateral caudate atrophy

Note. CSF = cerebrospinal fluid; DWI = diffusion-weighted imaging; FLAIR = fluid-attenuated inversion recovery; gad = gadolinium contrast; GE = gradient echo; MRA = magnetic resonance angiography; MRV = magnetic resonance venography; NPH = normal-pressure hydrocephalus.

Table 2–7. MRI results in 6,200 psychiatric inpatients: unexpected and potentially treatable findings

MRI finding	N	Percentage
Multiple sclerosis[a]	26	0.4
Hemorrhage	26	0.4
Temporal lobe cyst	22	0.4
Tumor	15	0.2
Vascular malformation	6	0.1
Hydrocephalus	4	0.1
Totals	99	**1.6**

[a]White matter abnormalities inferred as multiple sclerosis.
Source. Adapted from Rauch and Renshaw 1995.

Table 2–8. Summary of structural MRI study findings in schizophrenia (1988–2000)

Brain region	No. of studies	Percentage with positive findings	Percentage with negative findings
Whole brain	50	22	78
Lateral ventricles	55	80	20
Third ventricles	33	73	27
Fourth ventricle	5	20	80
Whole temporal lobe	51	61	39
Medial temporal lobe	49	74	26
Superior temporal gyrus, gray matter	12	100	0
Superior temporal gyrus, gray matter, and white matter	15	67	33
Planum temporale	10	60	40
Frontal lobe	50	60	40
Parietal lobe	15	60	40
Occipital lobe	9	44	56
Cerebellum	13	31	69
Basal ganglia	25	68	32
Thalamus	12	42	58
Corpus callosum	27	63	37
Cavum septum pellucidum	12	92	8

Source. Adapted from Shenton et al. 2001.

atric patient populations (e.g., poorly controlled bipolar disorder) (Soares and Mann 1997). The ultimate clinical significance of such findings is the subject of ongoing investigation and debate (Campbell and Coffey 2001).

There remain no pathognomonic structural MRI findings for primary psychiatric diseases (indeed, the search for such data has been a major driving force in the development of functional MRI in psychiatric neuroscience). However, a brief review of the literature in regard to the more common—albeit inconsistent—trends found in the structural imaging of psychiatric disease can help inform clinical efforts.

Schizophrenia

Interest in the neurobiology of schizophrenia was rekindled in the late 1970s, in large part due to CT studies of schizophrenia that provided initially compelling evidence that a substantial fraction of patients with schizophrenia had reduced cerebral volume, as revealed by enlarged ventricles and cortical sulci (confirming earlier pneumoencephalographic data) (Johnstone et al. 1976). These findings led to a proliferation of CT and subsequent MRI studies of schizophrenia (Shenton et al. 2001).

Beginning with one of the first MRI study of schizophrenia by Smith et al. in 1984, investigators have collected an impressive inventory of brain abnormalities in schizophrenia. Shenton et al. (2001) performed a comprehensive review and synthesis of structural MRI findings in schizophrenia, surveying almost 200 peer-reviewed MRI studies reported between 1988 and August 2000. Many of the schizophrenia-related brain abnormalities discovered by MRI converge with earlier postmortem findings.

In the Shenton et al. (2001) review, more frequent MRI findings in schizophrenia included ventricular en-

largement (80% of studies reviewed), cavum septum pellucidum (92% of studies reviewed), third-ventricle enlargement (73% of studies reviewed), and medial temporal abnormalities (74% of studies reviewed), including the amygdala, hippocampus, parahippocampal gyrus, and neocortical temporal regions (e.g., superior temporal gyrus in 100% of studies reviewed). Principal findings of Shenton and colleagues' review are summarized in Table 2–8.

A sample finding is illustrated in Figure 2–33. Note the enlarged lateral ventricles, increased CSF *(black)* in the left Sylvian fissure *(right side of scan),* increased CSF in the left temporal horn surrounding the left amygdala *(white arrow),* and tissue reduction in the left superior temporal gyrus in the patient with schizophrenia, compared with the healthy control subject (Shenton et al. 1992).

The timing of such abnormalities has not yet been determined. Many are evident in patients early in the disease course, suggesting that these structural changes do not entirely derive from disease progression (Shenton et al. 2001). Notwithstanding, there is evidence indi-

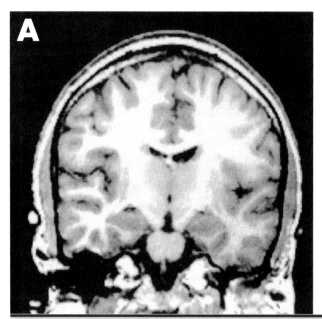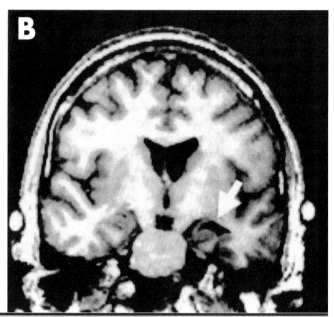

Figure 2–33.   Healthy control subject **(A)** and patient with schizophrenia **(B)** approximately anatomically co-registered, as seen on coronal T1-weighted MRI.

Source.   Reprinted from Shenton ME, Kikinis R, Jolesz FA, et al.: "Abnormalities of the Left Temporal Lobe and Thought Disorder in Schizophrenia. A Quantitative Magnetic Resonance Imaging Study." *New England Journal of Medicine* 327:604-612, 1992. Copyright 1992, The Massachusetts Medical Society. Used with permission.

cating that at least a subset of pathological features are progressive (Shenton et al. 2001).

Iatrogenic influences can complicate interpretation of MRI findings. For example, enlargement of the caudate volume has been reported early in the course of illness, but multiple studies suggest that this enlargement may be secondary to treatment with dopamine receptor antagonists (i.e., neuroleptics). Data supporting neuropathological changes over time in schizophrenia are summarized in Table 2–9.

Affective Disorders

Although there are no pathognomonic structural MRI findings as yet associated with affective disorders, a complex and inconsistent variety of structural MRI–discernible changes have been reported.

Data suggesting smaller volumes of the frontal lobes, amygdala, caudate, putamen, hippocampus, and cerebellum have been reported in some populations of patients with unipolar recurrent major depression (Renshaw and Parow 2002). On the basis of these observations, neuroanatomic models of mood regulation involving specific frontosubcortical circuits have been proposed for research using functional imaging techniques.

In patients with bipolar disorder, the most commonly reported findings have been increased white matter hyperintensities (Stoll et al. 2000) and enlarged ventricles (especially third), although it should be noted that the latter finding is controversial (Stoll et al. 2000). Select regional volume changes (e.g., prefrontal, temporal, cerebellar) have been less frequently reported (Drevets et al. 1997; Renshaw and Parow 2002; Soares and Mann 1997).

Obsessive-Compulsive Disorder

Because of theoretical models implicating caudate involvement and an early report of right caudate enlargement in patients with obsessive-compulsive disorder (OCD) (Scarone et al. 1992), several MRI studies of OCD have focused on the basal ganglia and frontostriatal circuits (Saxena et al. 1998). Evidence suggesting an association between striatal structural pathology and OCD includes an early report by Weilburg et al. (1989) of a patient with OCD whose MRI demonstrated left caudate atrophy and a left putamen cavitary lesion.

Support for structural MRI reports associating caudate pathology with OCD has come from multiple functional neuroimaging investigations of OCD. Nevertheless, structural MRI fails to reveal specific pathology in the majority of OCD patients.

Table 2–9. MRI studies of progressive volume changes in schizophrenia

Patient sample	Study	N	Region of interest	Follow-up period	Findings
First-episode schizophrenia	Chakos et al. 1994	21	Caudate	18 months	Increased caudate volume with typical antipsychotics; volume correlated with dose, inversely correlated with age at onset
Schizophrenia	Chakos et al. 1995	15	Caudate	12 months	Reduced caudate volume with atypical antipsychotics
Chronic schizophrenia	Corson et al. 1999	19	Caudate, lenticular nucleus	2 years	Typical antipsychotics increased size of caudate, lenticular nucleus; atypical antipsychotics decreased size
First-episode schizophrenia	Degreef et al. 1991	13	Cortical volume, ventricular volume	1–2 years	No difference in rate of change
First-episode schizophrenia	DeLisi et al. 1992	50	Temporal lobes, ventricular volume	2 years	No difference in temporal lobe or ventricular volume
First-episode schizophrenia	DeLisi et al. 1995	20	Cerebral hemispheres, medial temporal lobe, temporal lobe, lateral ventricles, caudate nucleus, corpus callosum	4 years	Rate of change greater in patients for left lateral ventricle
First-episode schizophrenia	DeLisi et al. 1997	50	Cerebral hemispheres, medial temporal lobe, lateral ventricles, cerebellum, caudate, corpus callosum, Sylvian fissure	≥4 years	Rate of change greater in patients for left and right hemispheres, right cerebellum, corpus callosum, and ventricles
First-episode schizophrenia	DeLisi et al. 1998	50	Cerebral hemisphere ventricles	5 years	Larger ventricles at baseline correlated with poorer premorbid functioning; larger ventricles at baseline also showed less of an increase in size at follow-up, compared with smaller ventricles at baseline
First-episode schizophrenia	Gur et al. 1998	20	Whole-brain CSF, frontal lobes, temporal lobes	2–3 years	Rate of change of frontal lobe volume increased; reduction in temporal lobe volume
Chronic schizophrenia	Gur et al. 1998	20	Whole-brain CSF, frontal lobes, temporal lobes	2–3 years	Rate of change of frontal lobe volume increased; reduction in temporal lobe volume
Childhood-onset schizophrenia	Jacobsen et al. 1998	10	Cerebral volume; superior, anterior temporal lobe; amygdala; hippocampus	2 years	Rate of change of total cerebral volume and temporal lobe structures increased in schizophrenia
First-episode psychosis	Keshavan et al. 1998	17	Cerebral volume, superior temporal gyrus, cerebellum	1 year	Volume of superior temporal gyrus inversely correlated with prodrome and psychosis duration; rate of change of superior temporal gyrus volume greater in patients; superior temporal gyrus volume enlarged with treatment in some patients (i.e., reversal of volume reduction after 1 year)

Table 2–9. MRI studies of progressive volume changes in schizophrenia *(continued)*

Patient sample	Study	N	Region of interest	Follow-up period	Findings
First-episode schizophrenia or schizoaffective disorder	Lieberman et al. 1996	62	Qualitative measure of lateral ventricles, third ventricle, frontal/parietal cortex, medial temporal lobe	18 months	Patients who had poor response to treatment showed more ventricular enlargement and reduced cortical volumes in comparison with patients who had better response to treatment
Childhood-onset schizophrenia	Rapoport et al. 1997	16	Ventricular volume; thalamic area; caudate nucleus; putamen; globus pallidus	2 years	Rate of change of ventricular volume and thalamic area increased in schizophrenia
Childhood-onset schizophrenia	Rapoport et al. 1999	15	Gray and white matter volume (frontal, temporal, parietal, occipital)	4 years	Rate of change of gray but not white matter in frontal, temporal, and parietal lobes increased in schizophrenia

Note. CSF=cerebrospinal fluid; MRI=magnetic resonance imaging.
Source. Adapted from Shenton ME, Dickey CC, Frumin M, et al.: "A Review of MRI Findings in Schizophrenia." *Schizophrenia Research* 49(1–2):1–52, 2001. Copyright 2001, Elsevier Science (www.elsevier.com). Used with permission.

A

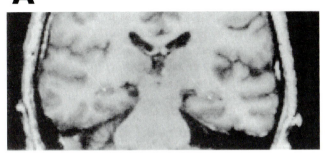

B

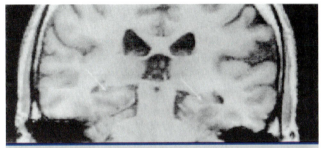

Figure 2–34. Patients (both combat veterans) with **(A)** and without **(B)** posttraumatic stress disorder, as seen on coronal T1-weighted MRI.
Source. Reprinted from Gurvits TV, Shenton ME, Hokama H, et al.: "Magnetic Resonance Imaging Study of Hippocampal Volume in Chronic Combat-Related Posttraumatic Stress Disorder." *Biological Psychiatry* 40:1091–1099, 1996. Copyright 1996, Elsevier Science (www.elsevier.com). Used with permission.

Posttraumatic Stress Disorder

Multiple studies have found moderate evidence for generalized cortical atrophy (e.g., sulcal widening) and specific hippocampal volume reduction (Figure 2–34) associated with severe long-standing posttraumatic stress disorder (PTSD). Intensive investigations are under way to better characterize these changes through functional neuroimaging.

Attention-Deficit/Hyperactivity Disorder

Many structural MRI studies of attention-deficit/hyperactivity disorder (ADHD) have been performed. Several have found smaller total brain volumes in ADHD subjects, representing an equal global reduction of gray and white matter (Rapoport et al. 2001). A sampling of subcortical structural MRI findings in ADHD are summarized in Table 2–10.

Longitudinal studies suggest that these changes in ADHD are fixed rather than progressive (Rapoport et al. 2001). Many of these findings support theoretical models of ADHD mechanisms implicating frontostriatal circuits; cerebellar contributions are intriguing and require further theoretical refinement.

Borderline Personality Disorder

Borderline personality disorder is increasingly a target of functional neuroimaging research, and there have been scattered reports of structural abnormalities in patients with this disorder. In a structural MRI study comparing 25 borderline personality disorder patients with age-matched control subjects, Lyoo et al. (1998) found smaller frontal lobe volumes in the patients. Other reports have described inconsistent findings.

Cognitive Disorders

Neuroimaging can be an essential aid in determining the etiology of cognitive dysfunction. Both primary neurodegenerative dementias and secondary processes can have associated structural abnormalities potentially discernible by MRI. For secondary processes, epidemiological studies have found the likelihood of detecting a clinically significant but covert (i.e., no noncognitive signs or symptoms indicating a lesion's presence) structural lesion (e.g., neoplasm, subdural hematoma, normal-pressure hydrocephalus) to be approximately 5% (Freter et al. 1998; Van Crevel et al. 1999).

Although we discuss the following primary neurodegenerative (e.g., AD, Pick's disease) and secondary processes (e.g., vascular dementia, human immunodeficiency virus [HIV] encephalopathy) under the category of cognitive disorders, *it should be emphasized that because all of these diseases also have the potential to produce a full range of psychiatric manifestations, the relevant neuroimaging discussion equally applies to evaluating affective, delusional, hallucinatory, and other psychiatric clinical expressions of these processes.* For example, frontal and thalamic strokes are known to be frequently associated with a variety of affective disorders, with important laterality considerations.

Primary Neurodegenerative Processes

Alzheimer's Disease. Alzheimer's-associated structural changes potentially demonstrable on MRI include temporal, parietal, and generalized atrophy (Figure 2–35). Coronal T1 images are best for specifically evaluating hippocampal atrophy.

Table 2–10. Subcortical MRI abnormalities reported in attention-deficit/hyperactivity disorder (ADHD)

Brain region	Study	Findings
Basal ganglia	Aylward et al. 1996	Left globus pallidus volume smaller in ADHD
	Castellanos et al. 1996	Symmetry in prefrontal brain, caudate, globus pallidus significantly decreased in ADHD
	Filipek et al. 1997	Left caudate smaller in ADHD; right anterior superior white matter diminished; posterior white matter volumes decreased only in stimulant nonresponders
	Mataro et al. 1997	Right caudate larger in ADHD
Cerebellum	Berquin et al. 1998	Posterior inferior cerebellar vermis volume significantly smaller in ADHD
	Mostofsky et al. 1998	Posterior inferior cerebellar vermis significantly smaller in ADHD
	Castellanos et al. 2001	Posterior inferior cerebellar vermis volume significantly smaller in ADHD

Note. MRI=magnetic resonance imaging.
Source. Adapted from Rapoport JL, Castellanos FX, Gogate N, et al.: "Imaging Normal and Abnormal Brain Development: New Perspectives for Child Psychiatry." *Australian and New Zealand Journal of Psychiatry* 35:272–281, 2001. Copyright 2001, Blackwell Publishing. Used with permission.

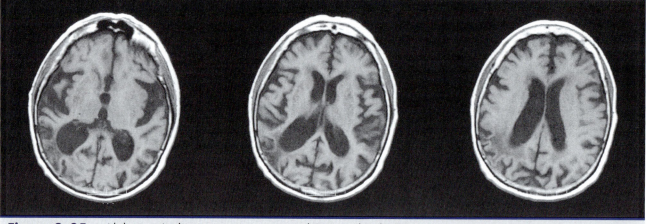

Figure 2–35. Alzheimer's disease as seen on axial T1-weighted MRI.

The hippocampus, parahippocampal gyrus, and temporal lobe in general are among brain regions most consistently implicated in neurodegenerative dementias, especially AD, even at an early stage (Scheltens 1999; Steffens et al. 2002). Neuropsychological assessments of recent memory are highly correlated with visually rated hippocampal atrophy, and hippocampal volume loss is strongly associated with neurofibrillary pathology in AD (Bobinski et al. 1996; Scheltens 1999).

Combining volumetric data with other potentially informative markers (e.g., apolipoprotein E genotyping, functional neuroimaging) may offer potential for improving diagnostic accuracy. For clinical purposes, volumetric measurements are helpful but are not required; visual inspection is usually sufficient.

Clinical studies of mild cognitive impairment, increasingly conceptualized as a harbinger of AD, have focused on early recognition to facilitate prompt intervention in an attempt to delay AD progression. Studies need to be performed to better characterize those structural imaging changes that are specifically associated with mild cognitive impairment, thus offering potential use as signifiers of future cognitive decline. However, given that atrophy is seen only after a substantial proportion of neurons have died, more sensitive methods (e.g., functional neuroimaging) for detecting such states will need to be developed for earlier diagnosis.

Frontotemporal Lobe Dementias. Structural neuroimaging usually—but not always—demonstrates bilateral and relatively symmetric frontal and/or temporal gyral atrophy in frontotemporal lobe dementias (FTLDs) (Gregory et al. 1999). This can be strikingly demonstrated on sagittal T1 images, especially medial sagittal

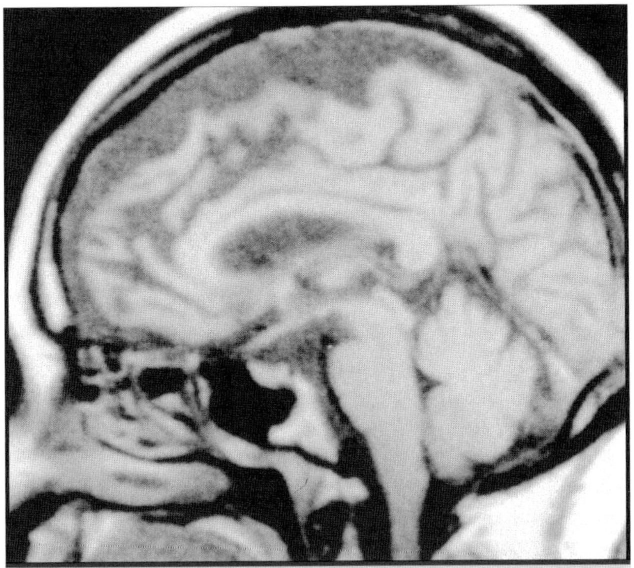

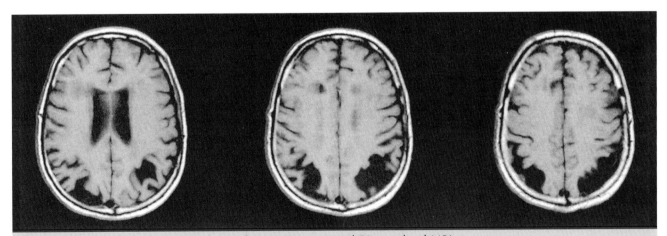

Figure 2–36. Frontotemporal lobar dementia as seen on sagittal T1-weighted MRI.

Source. Reprinted from Zimmerman RA, Gibby WA, Carmody RF (eds.): "The Aging Brain and Neurodegenerative Disorders," in *Neuroimaging: Clinical and Physical Principles.* New York, Springer, 2000, p. 960. Copyright 2000. Used with permission.

can show Sylvian fissure widening with atrophy of the insula, inferior frontal, and superior temporal lobes (dominant greater than nondominant hemisphere).

Dementia With Lewy Bodies. Nonspecific atrophy is the only typical MRI finding in dementia with Lewy bodies. Some patients show less temporal lobe atrophy than do patients with AD (Papka et al. 1998).

Posterior Cortical Atrophy. Posterior cortical atrophy is a selective lobar dementia characterized by initial disturbances of visual perception and integration (Benson et al. 1988). Involvement of the occipito-parietal region produces visuospatial and attentional disturbances (sometimes including Balint's syndrome), with relative sparing of personality, insight, and memory (Benson et al. 1988). Axial and sagittal T1 MR images can demonstrate the selective atrophy of posterior cortical structures (Figure 2–37).

Huntington's Disease. Huntington's disease is a prototypical subcortical neurodegenerative disorder, with multiple neuropsychiatric clinical manifestations. MRI findings, which are most discernible on coronal T1 images, include basal ganglia atrophy (primarily caudate).

images, which can reveal the "knife-edge" atrophy frequently seen at later stages of this disease (Miller and Gearhart 1999) (Figure 2–36).

In the semantic dementia variant of FTLD, MRI can reveal anterior temporal neocortical atrophy, with inferior and middle temporal gyri predominantly affected (Miller and Gearhart 1999). Asymmetries of temporal involvement can reflect relative severity of impairment for verbal versus visual concepts (word meaning versus object recognition) (Miller and Gearhart 1999). In the progressive nonfluent aphasia variant of FTLD, MRI

Secondary Processes

Structural

Normal-Pressure Hydrocephalus. The neuroradiological correlate of the clinical syndrome of normal-pressure hydrocephalus (classically marked by the triad of mental status change, gait apraxia, and urinary incontinence) is communicating (also called nonobstructive) hydrocephalus. It can often be challenging to distinguish genuine communicating hydrocephalus from

Figure 2–37. Posterior cortical atrophy as seen on axial T1-weighted MRI.

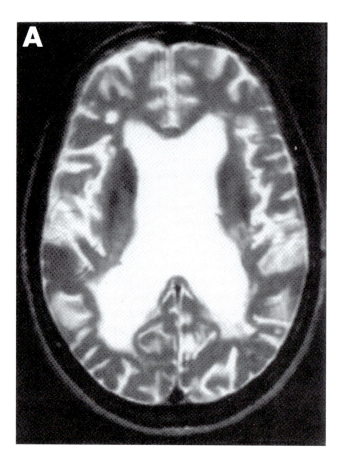

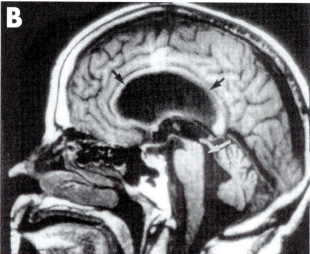

Figure 2–38. Normal-pressure hydrocephalus as seen on axial T2-weighted MRI **(A)** and sagittal T1-weighted MRI **(B)**.

ventricular dilatation proportionate to cerebral atrophy (hydrocephalus ex vacuo). Features supporting an interpretation of communicating hydrocephalus include ventricular enlargement disproportionate to cortical sulci depth, anterior third ventricle enlargement, bowing of the corpus callosum, and a flow void in the fourth ventricle on T2-weighted MRI (Figure 2–38) (Hurley et al. 1999).

Subdural Hematoma. Subdural hematoma can often be visualized on MRI as an extraneuraxial crescent-shaped abnormality. Typically involving a portion of—or, less commonly, an entire—cerebral convexity, subdural hematoma can also occur below tentorial dural regions. When subdural hematoma is convexity-based, ipsilateral obliteration of cortical sulci is usually seen (Figure 2–39). If the hematoma is large, mass effects such as ventricular compression can occur. It should be emphasized that subdural hematoma, particularly in the elderly, can present solely as a mental status change.

Metabolic

Wilson's Disease. In Wilson's disease, MRI often demonstrates bilateral cortical and basal ganglia abnormalities, including atrophy, with compensatory ventricular dilatation (Nazer et al. 1993; Thomas et al. 1993). Inconsistently present but relatively unique characteristics visualized on structural neuroimaging include basal ganglia cystic degeneration and cavitary necrosis.

Hepatic Encephalopathy. MRI findings in hepatic encephalopathy can include generalized atrophy and basal ganglia T1 hyperintensities (Maeda et al. 1997). The latter phenomenon appears to be in part secondary to deposition of paramagnetic substances (e.g., manganese) (Figure 2–40).

Toxic

Alcoholism. Chronic alcoholism can be associated with cerebellar (especially vermis) and generalized atrophy. Wernicke-Korsakov syndrome can be associated with mammillary body, thalamic, and midbrain abnormalities (e.g., FLAIR hyperintensities) (Figure 2–41).

Cerebrovascular

Strokes—small and large, ischemic and hemorrhagic, cortical and subcortical—represent the second most common cause of cognitive dysfunction, and laterality has long been known to have implications for affective function (e.g., association of left-hemisphere infarcts with depression and right-hemisphere infarcts with manic-like symptoms) (Robinson 1998).

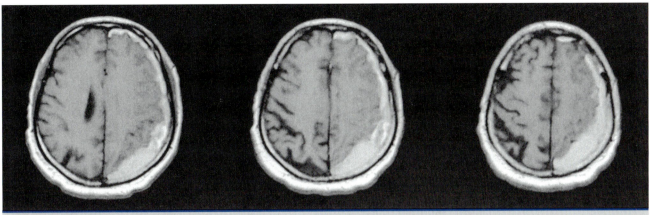

Figure 2–39. Subdural hematoma as seen on axial T1-weighted postcontrast MRI.

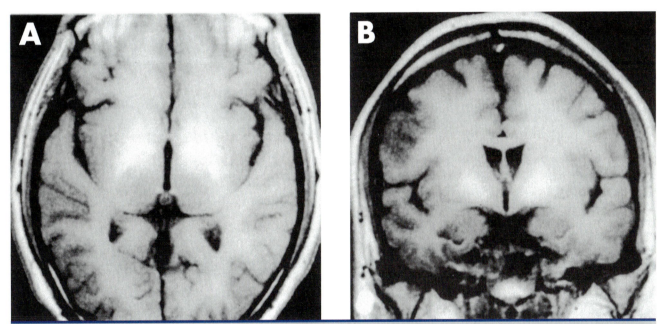

Figure 2–40. Hepatic encephalography (note basal ganglia hyperintensities) as seen on axial T1-weighted MRI **(A)** and coronal T1-weighted MRI **(B).**
Source. Reprinted from Maeda H, Sato M, Yoshikawa A, et al.: "Brain MR Imaging in Patients With Hepatic Cirrhosis: Relationship Between High Intensity Signal in Basal Ganglia on T1-Weighted Images and Elemental Concentrations in Brain." *Neuroradiology* 39:546–550, 1997. Copyright 1997, Springer-Verlag Heidelberg. Used with permission.

One of the most important uses of FLAIR MRI is for distinguishing subcortical and cortical ischemic disease in the differential diagnosis of cortical versus subcortical dysfunction. Cortical infarcts can be distinguished from subcortical ischemic disease, and subcortical disease can be separated into gray matter (e.g., basal ganglia) lesions and white matter lesions. Moreover, white matter disease can be further subdivided, with critical implications for neuropsychiatric function. For example, periventricular white matter disease (e.g., consistent with small-vessel pathology secondary to long-standing chronic hypertensive disease) can be distinguished from more extensive deep white matter pathology (e.g., consistent with more malignant cerebrovascular hypertension). Multiple small infarctions of subcortical white matter pathways, disconnecting circuitry among cognitively important cortical and subcortical centers, causes a subcortical microvascular leukoencephalopathy previously known as Binswanger's disease. MRI can also be invaluable in helping to diagnose syndromes that, although relatively rare, can produce prominent psychiatric symptoms (e.g., mitochondrial encephalopathy lactic acidosis and stroke [MELAS]). Sample MR images of cerebrovascular disease are presented in Figure 2–42.

Neoplastic

MRI is the gold standard for detecting primary and metastatic tumors (Figure 2–43). Even slow-growing benign tumors (e.g., meningioma), especially in frontal locations, can sometimes have psychiatric symptoms as their sole clinical expression (Lampl et al. 1995). Leptomeningeal disease can also be visualized as weaving of contrast enhancement into the sulci. Paraneoplastic limbic encephalitis can sometimes be visualized on FLAIR images, especially as medial temporal hyperintensities (Gultekin et al. 2000).

Radiation Necrosis

MRI often demonstrates leukoencephalopathy in patients who have undergone radiation therapy of the brain as treatment for intracranial malignancies (Figure 2–44). This effect can be delayed—in pathogenesis, clinical expression, and neuroradiological manifestations—for many years after treatment delivery.

Inflammatory

Multiple Sclerosis.   MRI greatly facilitates the diagnosis of multiple sclerosis. FLAIR images are especially useful, and sagittal FLAIR images in particular can be essential for diagnosis, because multiple sclerosis–related white matter plaques tend to originate pericallosally with medial centrifugal radiation, creating a characteristic pattern known as *Dawson's fingers* (Figure 2–45). Demonstration of this pattern, best observed with a sagittal orientation, helps differentiate such lesions from the multiple other causes (frequently benign and/or idiopathic) of white matter lesions visualized on FLAIR.

Neurosarcoidosis.   Central nervous system (CNS) sarcoidosis can manifest as nodular leptomeningeal enhancement and/or multifocal parenchymal lesions, including hypothalamic involvement. Neurosarcoidosis is also included in the wide differential diagnosis of subcortical T2 hyperintensities.

Infectious

Lyme Disease.   Lyme disease can be associated with variable primarily subcortical abnormalities, which are best visualized by FLAIR images.

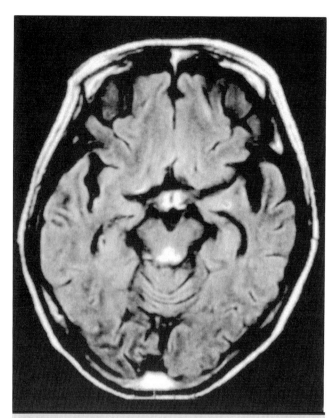

Figure 2–41. Alcoholism complicated by Wernicke-Korsakov syndrome, as seen on axial FLAIR MRI.
Source.   Reprinted from Chu K, Kang DW, Kim HJ, et al.: "Diffusion-Weighted Imaging Abnormalities in Wernicke Encephalopathy: Reversible Cytotoxic Edema?" *Archives of Neurology* 59:123–127, 2002. Copyright 2002, American Medical Association. Used with permission.

Neurosyphilis.   Tertiary syphilis can manifest in the CNS as a meningovascular inflammation, producing variable cortical and, more commonly, subcortical FLAIR-detectable lesions.

Herpes Encephalitis.   In herpes encephalitis, MRI can reveal temporal lobe pathology—including loss of gray–white differentiation, edema, hemorrhagic components, and/or abnormal contrast enhancement (Figure 2–46)—during the first week of disease (Schroth et al. 1987).

Human Immunodeficiency Virus.   Multiple potential primary (e.g., nonspecific atrophy) and secondary (e.g., opportunistic infections) HIV-related pathologies can be visualized on MRI (Figure 2–47).

Creutzfeldt-Jakob Disease.   MRI often demonstrates a characteristic "cortical ribboning" on diffusion-weighted imaging (Figure 2–48).

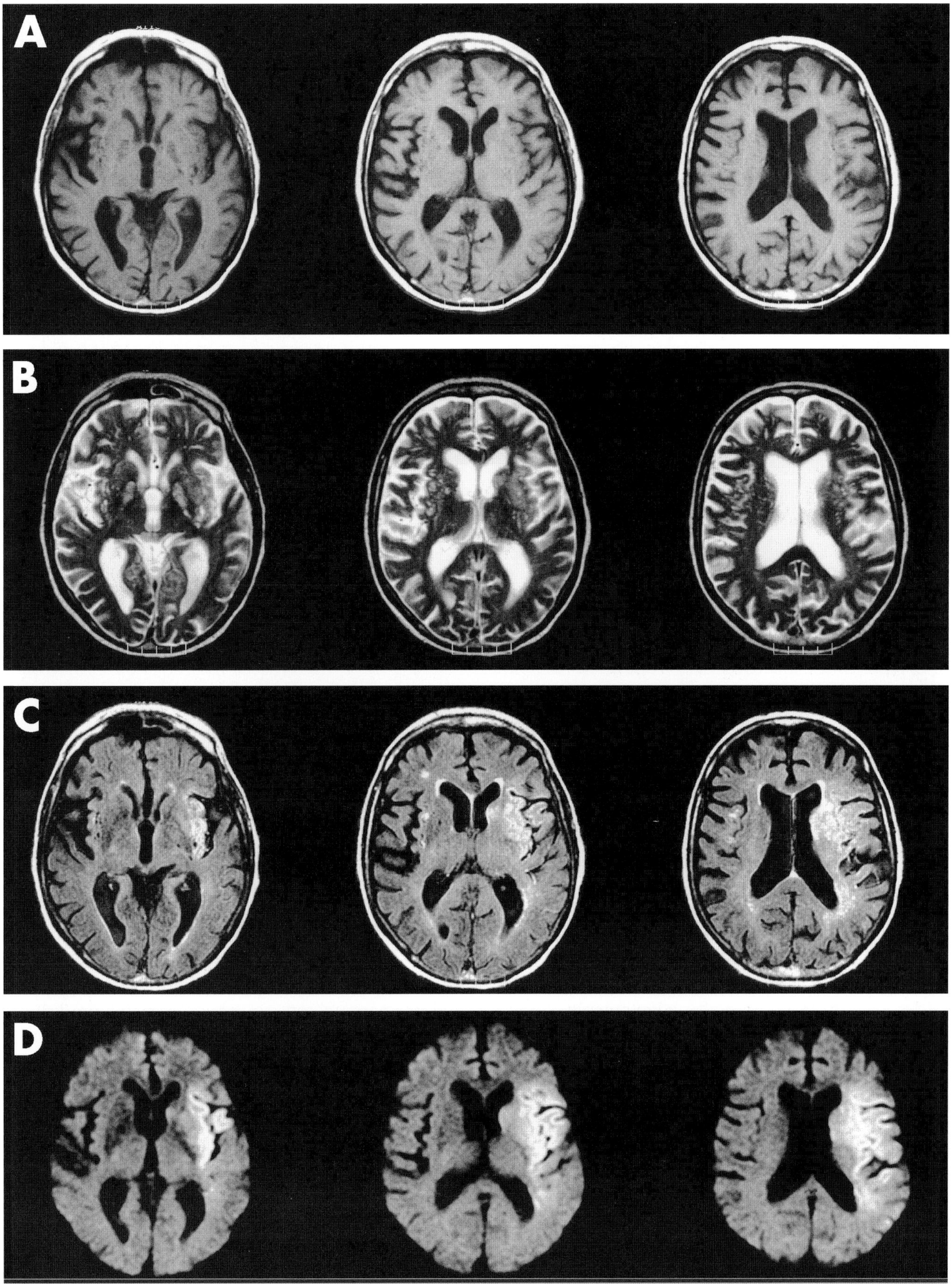

Figure 2–42. Cerebrovascular disease as seen on axial T1-weighted MRI **(A)**, axial T2-weighted MRI **(B)**, axial FLAIR MRI **(C)**, and axial DWI MRI **(D).**

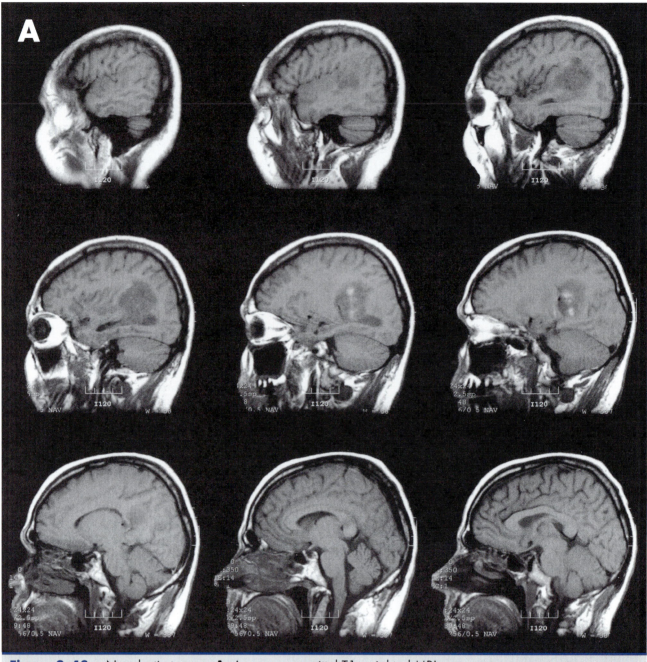

Figure 2–43. Neoplastic tumors. **A,** As seen on sagittal T1-weighted MRI.

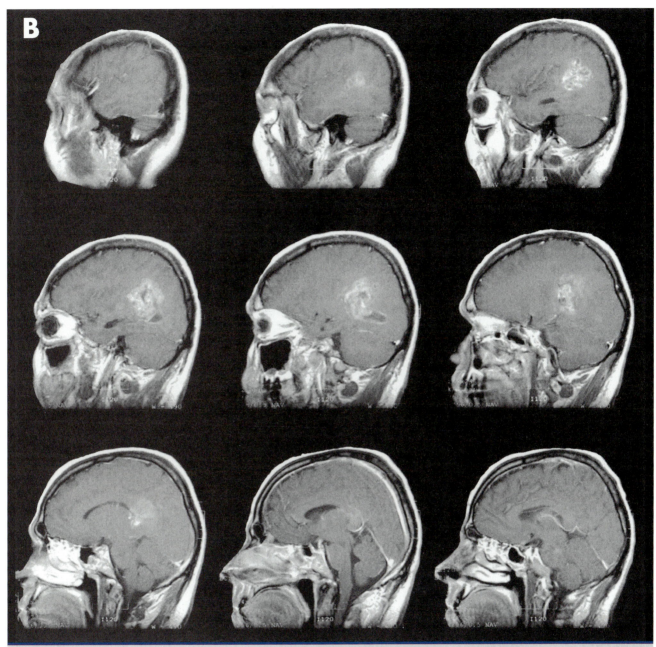

Figure 2–43 (continued). Neoplastic tumors. **B,** As seen on sagittal T1-weighted postcontrast MRI.

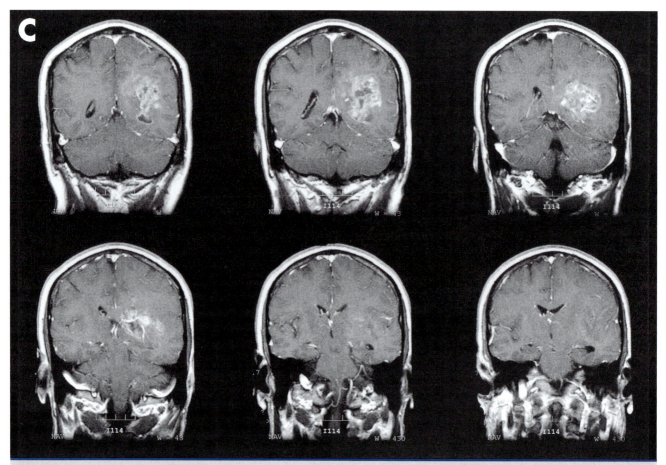

Figure 2–43 (continued). Neoplastic tumors. **C,** As seen on coronal T1-weighted postcontrast MRI.

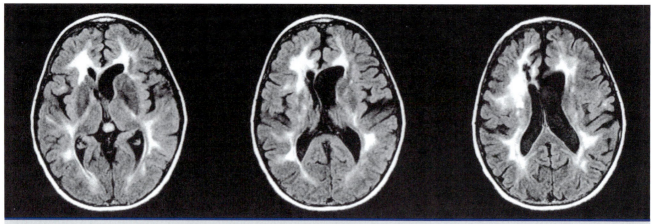

Figure 2–44. Radiation necrosis as seen on axial FLAIR MRI.

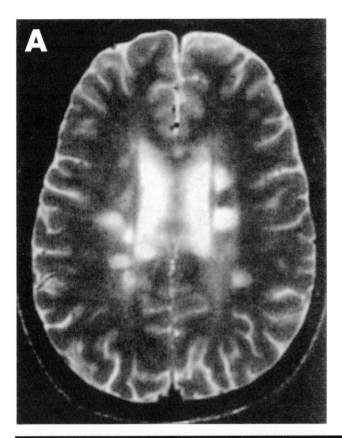

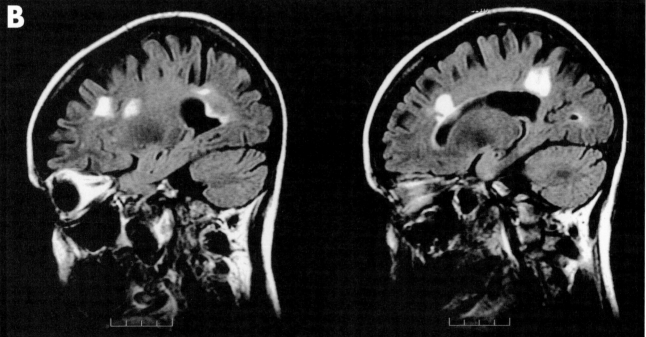

Figure 2–45. Multiple sclerosis as seen on axial T2-weighted MRI **(A)** and revealing Dawson's fingers on sagittal FLAIR MRI **(B).**

Source. Image A reprinted from Loevner LA: *Brain Imaging.* St. Louis, MO, CV Mosby, 1999, p. 27. Copyright 1999, Elsevier Science Inc. (www.elsevier.com). Used with permission.

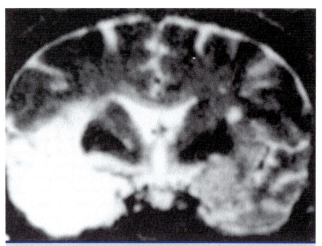

Figure 2–46.   Herpes simplex encephalitis as seen on coronal T2-weighted MRI.

Source.   Reprinted from Schroth G, Gawehn J, Thron A, et al.: "Early Diagnosis of Herpes Simplex Encephalitis by MRI." *Neurology* 37:179–183, 1987. Copyright 1987, Lippincott Williams & Wilkins (www.lww.com). Used with permission.

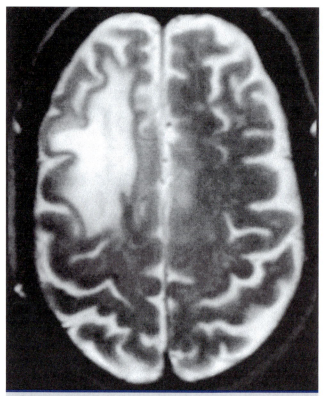

Figure 2–47.   HIV-related leukoencephalopathy (progressive multifocal leukoencephalopathy) as seen on axial T2-weighted MRI.

Source.   Reprinted from Loevner LA: *Brain Imaging.* St. Louis, MO, CV Mosby, 1999, p. 89. Copyright 1999, Elsevier Science Inc. (www. elsevier.com). Used with permission.

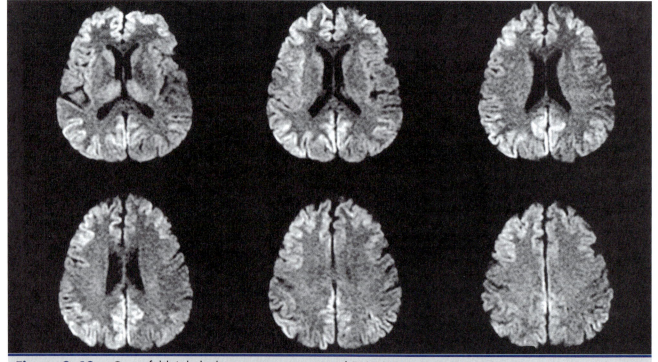

Figure 2–48.   Creutzfeldt-Jakob disease as seen on axial DWI MRI.

Clinical Indications: When to Order an MRI

Relatively few studies have substantiated the utility of MRI for the evaluation of brain pathology in patients with primary psychiatric illness. *No formal psychiatric practice guidelines exist for when to obtain an MRI.* As with all diagnostic modalities, assessing the clinical value and cost-effectiveness of any diagnostic test is methodologically complex. Because MRI is generally well tolerated by patients and involves few known risks, the disadvantages of performing an MRI (other than cost) would seem to be few. However, other potential clinical disadvantages exist. With MR imaging power, incidental findings (e.g., clinically insignificant punctate white matter lesions) are not uncommon; MRI's greater sensitivity comes at the price of some specificity for differentiating pathology from clinically insignificant findings (e.g., white matter T2 hyperintensities). Thus, costs of false-positive findings resulting in unnecessary follow-up investigations (e.g., lumbar puncture) must also be considered.

The management decision-making value of an MRI can be conceptualized in terms of its potential to alter treatment and therefore presumably outcome (Rauch and Renshaw 1995). Some authors have therefore argued that to the extent that a psychiatric disorder attributable to either primary or secondary MRI-evident CNS pathology would be treated in the same way as symptoms derived from a primary psychiatric etiology, clarifying a CNS process causing the clinical phenomenon, in cases where the CNS process does not itself have a specific treatment, is of limited management value. However, other investigators and clinicians claim that confirming a diagnosis with higher certainty by ruling out "organic disease" can have important prognostic implications, as well as difficult-to-quantify psychological value, especially in the case of new-onset psychiatric disease. Of course, this also raises the issue of what constitutes "organic disease"— a concept gradually becoming indistinct with theoretical and technological development.

Improved data defining clinical risk factors for that subset of psychiatric patients who would benefit from neuroimaging would aid in optimizing the cost-effectiveness of MRI. Candidate risk factors include advanced age, history of head trauma, presence of cognitive deficits, and abnormalities on neurological examination (Rauch and Renshaw 1995).

Table 2–11 presents an amalgam of heuristics regarding commonly accepted clinical indications for ordering an MRI combined with the authors' collective clinical experience as consulting neuropsychiatrists and behavioral neurologists. These recommendations do not supplant established practice guidelines for neuroimaging of primary neurological disease states. Instead, they are meant to be applied in the context of clinical evaluation of primary or comorbid psychiatric phenomena.

We recommend screening structural neuroimaging before ECT when the neurological history is marked by or the examination yields features suggesting the possibility of intracranial pathology with potential for ECT-related complications (e.g., mass-related increased intracranial pressure, aneurysm-related hemorrhage). For spinal taps, given that most diagnostic indications for performing lumbar puncture in psychiatry potentially involve associated MRI findings, it is difficult to imagine a clinical scenario in which a lumbar puncture would be indicated but an MRI would not. Furthermore, because ascertaining absence of any cause for raised intracranial pressure is an essential prerequisite to performing a lumbar puncture, and because neuroimaging is the only way other than quality fundoscopy to confirm such absence, MRI represents an effective means of satisfying all of these diagnostic mandates.

How to Order an MRI: Ensuring That the Images Needed to Answer the Diagnostic Question Are Acquired

If no image types are specified, the MRI protocol (i.e., which pulse sequences and slice orientations will be used) is determined by a neuroradiologist on the basis of information provided in the clinical referral. Thus, the more detail contained in the referral query, the greater the likelihood that the images needed to resolve the diagnostic issue in question will in fact be obtained. For example, properly imaging a patient with a cancer history requires pre- and postcontrast images to be obtained to rule out CNS neoplastic involvement; imaging a patient as part of an evaluation for memory dysfunction should include coronal images obtained to facilitate hippocampal evaluation; and so on. Thus, *attention to the known pathophysiologies of processes being considered in the differential diagnosis should inform construction of the image acquisition protocol.*

Table 2–11. Relative indications for ordering an MRI

Indication	Example(s)
History	
Congenital/developmental	Perinatal complications
	Congenital CNS anomaly
	Learning disorder
	Febrile seizure history
Disease course characteristics	Acute-onset signs/symptoms
	Rapidly progressive signs/symptoms
	Treatment-refractory signs/symptoms
	Atypically late-onset signs/symptoms
Risk factors	Head trauma
	Significant/long-standing hypertension
	Endocrine disease (e.g., diabetes, hypothyroidism)
	Neoplastic disease
	Potential toxin exposure
	CNS-affecting autoimmune disease
	CNS-penetrable infectious disease
CNS signs	
Global consciousness or sensorium disturbances	Delirium
	Catatonia
Neurobehavioral/cognitive deficit(s) disproportionate to typical cognitive epiphenomena of primary psychiatric disturbance	Receptive language dysfunction
	Expressive language dysfunction
	Objective memory impairment
	Visuospatial dysfunction
	Focal executive dysfunction
Focal elementary neurological deficit(s)	Cranial nerve palsy
	Focal motor deficit
	Dysmetria
	Movement disorder
	Focal sensory deficit
	Gait disturbance
Symptoms	New hallucinations
	New onset or change in quality/frequency of headaches
	New dizziness and/or vertigo
	Visual change
	Hearing change
	New focal weakness/numbness/paresthesias
	Excessive somnolence
	Extreme apathy

Note. CNS=central nervous system.

When a CT Is Acceptable or Even Preferred

The imaging modality of first choice for initial evaluation of any acute clinical change potentially attributable to intracranial pathology remains a noncontrast head CT. CT is quick, widely available, relatively inexpensive, and provides imaging data informing almost any clinical condition requiring *urgent* intervention, including mass effect, herniation, hydrocephalus, and hemorrhage. The only exception is when acute ischemic injury is suspected and DWI MRI is readily available, because acute ischemic stroke is not well visualized on CT. Because contrast shows up as bright hyperdensity on CT, noncontrast examination is preferred as the initial study, given that contrast could obscure acute hemorrhage, which also appears as bright hyperdensity.

In nonacute settings, CT may still have certain advantages. CT is faster (although image acquisition speed of MRI is increasingly approaching that of CT), and the CT scanner is less narrow and deep than MRI scanners, making CT more easily tolerated by patients with claustrophobia. Even with GE MRI, CT is better for evaluating acute bleeding. CT is preferred for detecting calcifications and evaluating skull fractures (especially at the base of the skull). CT remains cheaper, and of course, CT is mandated when intracranial imaging is required and the patient has an absolute contraindication to MRI.

That said, MRI is superior in almost all other ways (e.g., overall resolution, gray–white differentiation, white matter lesion detection, multiplanar imaging). For evaluating the posterior fossa and brain stem, even CT's acute advantages become relatively nullified, given that CT images can become degraded by dense bone artifact streaking.

Contraindications to MRI

Because MRI does not involve ionizing radiation, it is generally considered to be among the safest of imaging modalities. However, the magnetic fields generated are strong and getting stronger as higher-powered magnets are becoming available. Foreign objects that can be affected by these magnetic fields constitute a contraindication to MRI. Ferromagnetic objects can be vulnerable to movement (potentially causing structural injury), current conduction (potentially causing electrical shock), heating (possibly causing burn injury), and artifact generation. Cardiac pacemakers can malfunction, in addition to the potential for structural, electrical, and heat-related complications (Shellock 2001). Metal cerebral aneurysm clips also represent an absolute contraindication. Because some tattoos contain metallic pigments, even these can constitute a relative contraindication in higher–field strength MRI scanners (i.e., ≥ 3 tesla). Equipment with ferromagnetic components is also prohibited from the scanner suite. For example, MRI is contraindicated for patients with attached medical devices such as intravenous pumps, cardiac monitors (including Holter monitors), and ventilators (MRI-safe ventilators are manufactured but are relatively scarce). Certain vagal nerve stimulators are MRI-safe, but this needs to be explicitly clarified on an individual basis. With the expansion of MRI use, a growing number of implanted medical devices are being made MRI-safe. Lists of MRI-safe and MRI-unsafe devices are available and are periodically updated. These guidelines are summarized in Table 2–12.

Some metallic objects do not necessarily pose a health hazard, but can still nevertheless produce image artifacts (e.g., dental fillings, false eyelashes, hair bands).

No specific weight limit restrictions exist; however, because of associated girth complications, patients whose weight exceeds approximately 300 pounds are often unable to fit within the standard MRI scanner.

Table 2–12. Sample foreign bodies constituting potential contraindications to MRI

Contraindication level	Device or foreign object	Comments
Absolute	Cardiac pacemaker	
	Metallic heart valve containing ferromagnetic components	
	Porcine heart valves with metallic frames	Some frames are MRI-safe
	Aneurysm clips	Some new clips are MRI-safe
	Vagal nerve stimulator (VNS)	Some VNSs are MRI-safe
	Metallic cochlear implants	
	Any ferromagnetic-containing implant	
	Any foreign body whose composition is unknown	E.g., bullet fragments
Relative	Orthopedic implants	Most are now MRI-safe; consult a device list
	History of occupational exposure to metallic debris (e.g., welding)	Screen for history of accidents, especially eye injuries
	Permanent metallic body piercings	
	Tattoos	Only a problem in higher-strength magnets (e.g., ≥ 3 T)

Although probably quite safe, MRI is still considered to be relatively contraindicated during pregnancy. However, if intracranial pathology is suspected and a brain image is needed, MRI is much preferable to CT, given CT's attendant ionizing radiation exposure.

If there is any doubt regarding MR safety, the attending neuroradiologist or chief MRI technologist should be consulted *before* requisitioning an MRI. Rare but serious adverse events have occurred after non-MRI-safe objects have been discovered in patients already in the MRI scanner.

How to Prepare Patients for an MRI

After being "de-metallized" (i.e., removing all metal objects, including jewelry, magnetized cards, communication devices, earrings, and the like), the patient is placed supine on a gantry, which is then advanced into the scanner bore. Depth of placement in the MRI scanner depends on the body part being imaged; for brain MRIs, the patient is loaded head-first and advanced up to the lower torso. Scanning time varies according to protocol. An average MRI scanning session lasts approximately 30 minutes. However, a protocol requiring a large number of different sequences, fine cuts through a specific region (e.g., pituitary protocol), and/or postcontrast images can extend scanning time beyond an hour.

MRI scanner bores are usually 2 to 3 feet wide and several feet deep. Being placed within this space often produces a sense of confinement. Given the loud, harsh noises of the machine, the requirement to remain still, and the length of time required, many patients report significant anxiety, and a subset of these experience significant claustrophobia or frank panic attacks. Of course, for those patient populations with psychiatric disease potentially aggravated by the scanning experience (e.g., claustrophobia, anxiety disorders, PTSD), the percentages of patients unable to comply with an MRI are higher. For certain patients, fear of the scanning experience becomes an exclusionary factor. Some of these patients can be made sufficiently comfortable by means of premedication. Also, minimizing scanning time by ordering only those images that are needed, excluding imaging sequences that are not required to answer the diagnostic query, can bring the scanning experience into a tolerable time range.

Premedication

Oral administration of a rapid-onset, short-acting benzodiazepine or other sedative agent 30 minutes to 1 hour before scanning is usually effective in preventing claustrophobia-related anxiety reactions. In children, antihistamines (e.g., diphenhydramine) or, more rarely, chloral hydrate are used. In rare circumstances, intravenous sedation in the scanning room can be administered to permit acquisition of a clinically crucial MRI for a patient who is otherwise unable to tolerate scanning or who is without capacity to remain sufficiently still.

Open and Stand-Up MRI

Although improving, many currently operational open and stand-up MRI systems produce images of lower quality than their closed-configured counterparts. Because pathology causing neuropsychiatric symptoms can be subtle, we recommend the higher-resolution images produced by closed systems. Of course, for patients with severe claustrophobia resistant to anxiolytic premedication (or patients for whom such agents are contraindicated), open MR images are sometimes the only ones attainable.

When and Where to Refer Patients With Abnormal MRI Findings

Any clinically significant newly discovered intracranial abnormality unrelated to a primary psychiatric syndrome should prompt referral of the patient to a neurologist for further evaluation. Findings with potential for rapidly serious complication (e.g., expanding subdural hematoma) warrant urgent referral for appropriate management (e.g., to the emergency department). Because for many patients the MRI scan you order is their first neuroradiological examination, a significant number of incidental findings can be expected. Direct discussion with the interpreting neuroradiologist can often clarify the clinical implications of more subtle findings. MRI's remarkable in vivo brain-imaging capacity fosters a multidisciplinary approach to patient management.

References

Aylward EH, Reiss AL, Reader MJ, et al: Basal ganglia volumes in children with attention-deficit hyperactivity disorder. J Child Neurol 11:112–115, 1996

Benson DF, Davis RJ, Snyder BD: Posterior cortical atrophy. Arch Neurol 45:789–793, 1988

Berquin PC, Giedd JN, Jacobsen LK, et al: Cerebellum in attention-deficit hyperactivity disorder: a morphometric MRI study. Neurology 50:1087–1093, 1998

Bertelson JA, Price BH: Depression and psychosis in neurological practice, in Neurology in Clinical Practice. Edited by Bradley WG, Daroff RB, Fenichel GM, et al. Philadelphia, PA, Elsevier, 2003, pp 103–116

Bobinski M, Wegiel J, Wisniewski HM, et al: Neurofibrillary pathology—correlation with hippocampal formation atrophy in Alzheimer's disease. Neurobiol Aging 17:909–919, 1996

Campbell JJ, Coffey CE: Neuropsychiatric significance of subcortical hyperintensity. J Neuropsychiatry Clin Neurosci 13:261–288, 2001

Castellanos FX, Giedd JN, Marsh WL, et al: Quantitative brain magnetic resonance imaging in attention-deficit hyperactivity disorder. Arch Gen Psychiatry 53:607–616, 1996

Castellanos FX, Giedd JN, Berquin PC, et al: Quantitative brain magnetic resonance imaging in girls with attention deficit hyperactivity disorder. Arch Gen Psychiatry 58:289–295, 2001

Chakos MH, Lieberman JA, Bilder RM, et al: Increase in caudate nuclei volumes of first episode schizophrenic patients taking antipsychotic drugs. Am J Psychiatry 151:1430–1436, 1994

Chakos MH, Lieberman JA, Alvir J, et al: Caudate nuclei volumes in schizophrenic patients treated with typical antipsychotics or clozapine (letter). Lancet 345:456–457, 1995

Corson PW, Nopoulos P, Miller DD, et al: Change in basal ganglia volume over 2 years in patients with schizophrenia: typical versus atypical neuroleptics. Am J Psychiatry 156:1200–1204, 1999

Degreef G, Ashtari M, Wu HW, et al: Follow up MRI study in first episode schizophrenia. Schizophr Res 5:204–206, 1991

DeLisi LE, Stritzke P, Riordan H, et al: The timing of brain morphological changes in schizophrenia and their relationship to clinical outcome. Biol Psychiatry 31:241–254, 1992

DeLisi LE, Tew W, Xie S, et al: A prospective follow-up study of brain morphology and cognition in first-episode schizophrenic patients: preliminary findings. Biol Psychiatry 38:349–360, 1995

DeLisi LE, Sakuma M, Tew W, et al: Schizophrenia as a chronic brain process: a study of progressive brain structural change subsequent to the onset of schizophrenia. Psychiatry Res 74:129–140, 1997

DeLisi LE, Sakuma M, Ge S, et al: Association of brain structural change with the heterogeneous course of schizophrenia from early childhood through five years subsequent to a first hospitalization. Psychiatry Res 84:75–88, 1998

Drevets WC, Price JL, Simpson JR, et al: Subgenual prefrontal cortex abnormalities in mood disorders. Nature 386:824–827, 1997

Filipek PA, Semrud-Clikeman M, Steingard RJ, et al: Volumetric MRI analysis comparing subjects having attention-deficit hyperactivity disorder with normal controls. Neurology 48:589–601, 1997

Foong J, Maier M, Clark CA, et al: Neuropathologic abnormalities of the corpus callosum in schizophrenia: a diffusion tensor imaging study. J Neurol Neurosurg Psychiatry 68:242–244, 2000

Freter S, Bergman H, Gold S, et al: Prevalence of potentially reversible dementias and actual reversibility in a memory clinic cohort. CMAJ 159(6):657–662, 1998

Gregory CA, Serra-Mestres J, Hodges JR: Early diagnosis of the frontal variant of frontotemporal dementia: how sensitive are standard neuroimaging and neuropsychological tests? Neuropsychiatry Neuropsychol Behav Neurol 12:128–135, 1999

Gultekin SH, Rosenfeld MR, Voltz R, et al: Paraneoplastic limbic encephalitis: neurological symptoms, immunological findings, and tumor association. Brain 123(7):1481–1494, 2000

Gur RE, Cowell P, Turetsky BI, et al: A follow-up magnetic resonance imaging study of schizophrenia: relationship of neuroanatomical changes to clinical and neurobehavioral measures. Arch Gen Psychiatry 55:145–152, 1998

Hurley RA, Bradley WG Jr, Latifi HT, et al: Normal pressure hydrocephalus: significance of MRI in a potentially treatable dementia. J Neuropsychiatry Clin Neurosci 11:297–300, 1999

Innis RB, Malison RT: Principles of neuroimaging, in Comprehensive Textbook of Psychiatry, Edited by Kaplan H, Saddock B. Baltimore, MD, Williams & Wilkins, 1995, pp 89–103

Jacobsen LK, Giedd JN, Castellanos FX, et al: Progressive reduction of temporal lobe structures in childhood-onset schizophrenia. Am J Psychiatry 155:678–685, 1998

Johnstone EC, Crow TJ, Frith CD, et al: Cerebral ventricular size and cognitive impairment in chronic schizophrenia. Lancet 2(7992):924–926, 1976

Kandel ER, Schwartz JH, Jessell TM (eds): Principles of Neural Science, 4th Edition. New York, McGraw-Hill, 2000

Keshavan MS, Haas GL, Kahn CE, et al: Superior temporal gyrus and the course of early schizophrenia: progressive, static, or reversible? J Psychiatr Res 32:161–167, 1998

Klingberg T, Hedehus M, Temple E, et al: Microstructure of temporo-parietal white matter as a basis for reading ability: evidence from diffusion tensor magnetic resonance imaging. Neuron 25:493–500, 2000

Ketonen LM, Berg MJ: Clinical Neuroradiology. London, Arnold, 1997

Lampl Y, Barak Y, Achiron A, et al: Intracranial meningiomas: correlation of peritumoral edema and psychiatric disturbances. Psychiatry Res 58:177–180, 1995

Lieberman JA, Alvir JM, Koreen A, et al: Psychobiologic correlates of treatment response in schizophrenia. Neuropsychopharmacology 14:132–215, 1996

Lim KO, Hedehus M, Moseley M, et al: Compromised white matter tract integrity in schizophrenia inferred from diffusion tensor imaging. Arch Gen Psychiatry 56:367–374, 1999

Lufkin RB: The MRI Manual. St. Louis, MO, CV Mosby, 1998

Lyoo IK, Han MH, Cho DY: A brain MRI study in subjects with borderline personality disorder. J Affect Disord 50: 235–243, 1998

Maeda H, Sato M, Yoshikawa A, et al: Brain MR imaging in patients with hepatic cirrhosis: relationship between high intensity signal in basal ganglia on T1-weighted images and elemental concentrations in brain. Neuroradiology 39:546–550, 1997

Mataro M, Garcia-Sanchez C, Junque C, et al: Magnetic resonance imaging measurement of the caudate nucleus in adolescents with attention deficit hyperactivity disorder and its relationship with neuropsychological and behavioral measures. Arch Neurology 54:963–968, 1997

Miller BL, Gearhart R: Neuroimaging in the diagnosis of frontotemporal dementia. Dement Geriatr Cogn Disord 10 (suppl 1): 71–74, 1999

Mostofsky SH, Reiss AL, Lockart P, et al: Evaluation of cerebellar size in attention deficit hyperactivity disorder. J Child Neurology 13:434–439, 1998

Nazer H, Brismar J, al-Kawi MZ, et al: Magnetic resonance imaging of the brain in Wilson's disease. Neuroradiology 35:130–133, 1993

Papka M, Rubio A, Schiffer RB: A review of Lewy body disease, an emerging concept of cortical dementia. J Neuropsychiatry Clin Neurosci 10(3):267–279, 1998

Rapoport JL, Giedd JN, Blumenthal J, et al: Progressive cortical change during adolescence in childhood-onset schizophrenia: a longitudinal magnetic resonance imaging study. Arch Gen Psychiatry 56:649–654, 1999

Rapoport JL, Giedd JN, Kimra S, et al: Childhood-onset schizophrenia: progressive ventricular change during adolescence. Arch Gen Psychiatry 54:897–903, 1997

Rapoport JL, Castellanos FX, Gogate N, et al: Imaging normal and abnormal brain development: new perspectives for child psychiatry. Aust N Z J Psychiatry 35:272–281, 2001

Rauch SL, Renshaw PF: Clinical neuroimaging in psychiatry. Harv Rev Psychiatry 2:297–312, 1995

Renshaw PF, Parow AM: Psychiatric disease, in Magnetic Resonance Imaging of the Brain and Spine. Edited by Atlas SW. Philadelphia, PA, Lippincott, Williams & Wilkins, 2002, pp 1993–2019

Robinson RG: The Clinical Neuropsychiatry of Stroke: Cognitive, Behavioral and Emotional Disorders Following Vascular Brain Injury. Cambridge, UK, Cambridge University Press, 1998

Rose SE, Chen F, Chalk JB, et al: Loss of connectivity in Alzheimer's disease: an evaluation of white matter tract integrity with colour coded MR diffusion tensor imaging. J Neurol Neurosurg Psychiatry 69:528–530, 2000

Rugg-Gunn FJ, Symms MR, Barker GJ, et al: Diffusion imaging shows abnormalities after blunt head trauma when conventional magnetic resonance imaging is normal. J Neurol Neurosurg Psychiatry 70:530–533, 2001

Saxena S, Brody AL, Schwartz JM, et al: Neuroimaging and frontal-subcortical circuitry in obsessive-compulsive disorder. Br J Psychiatry Suppl (37):26–37, 1998

Scarone S, Colombo C, Livian S, et al: Increased right caudate nucleus size in obsessive compulsive disorder: detection with magnetic resonance imaging. Psychiatry Res 45:115–121, 1992

Scheltens P: Early diagnosis of dementia: neuroimaging. J Neurol 246:16–20, 1999

Schild HH: MRI Made Easy, 5th Edition. Berlin, Germany, Schering AG/Berlex Laboratories, 1999

Schroth G, Gawehn J, Thron A, et al: Early diagnosis of herpes simplex encephalitis by MRI. Neurology 37:179–183, 1987

Shellock FG: MR Procedures and Metallic Objects. Philadelphia, PA, Lippincott, Williams & Wilkins, 2001

Shenton ME, Kikinis R, Jolesz FA, et al: Abnormalities of the left temporal lobe and thought disorder in schizophrenia: a quantitative magnetic resonance imaging study. N Engl J Med 327:604–612, 1992

Shenton ME, Dickey CC, Frumin M, et al: A review of MRI findings in schizophrenia. Schizophr Res 49(1–2):1–52, 2001

Smith RC, Calderon M, Ravichandran GK, et al: Nuclear magnetic resonance in schizophrenia: a preliminary study. Psychiatry Res 12:137–147, 1984

Soares JC, Mann JJ: The anatomy of mood disorders—review of structural neuroimaging studies. Biol Psychiatry 41:86–106, 1997

Steffens DC, Payne ME, Greenberg DL, et al: Hippocampal volume and incident dementia in geriatric depression. Am J Geriatr Psychiatry 10:62–71, 2002

Stoll A, Renshaw P, Yurgelun-Todd D, et al: Neuroimaging in bipolar disorder. Biol Psychiatry 48:505–517, 2000

Taber KH, Pierpaoli C, Rose SE, et al: The future for diffusion tensor imaging in neuropsychiatry. J Neuropsychiatry Clin Neurosci 14:1–5, 2002

Thomas KA, Aquilonius SM, Bergstrom K, et al: Magnetic resonance imaging of the brain in Wilson's disease. Neuroradiology 35:134–141, 1993

Van Crevel H, van Gool WA, Walstra GJM: Early diagnosis of dementia: which tests are indicated? What are their costs? J Neurol 246:73–78, 1999

Weilburg JB, Mesulam MM, Weintraub S, et al: Focal striatal abnormalities in a patient with obsessive-compulsive disorder. Archives of Neurology 46:233–235, 1989

Werring DJ, Clark CA, Barker GJ, et al: The structural and functional mechanisms of motor recovery: complementary use of diffusion tensor and functional magnetic resonance imaging in a traumatic injury of the internal capsule. J Neurol Neurosurg 65:863–869, 1998

Suggested Readings

Baumann B, Bogerts B: The pathomorphology of schizophrenia and mood disorders: similarities and differences. Schizophr Res 39:141–148, 1999

Bremner JD: Alterations in brain structure and function associated with post-traumatic stress disorder. Semin Clin Neuropsychiatry 4:249–255, 1999a

Bremner JD: Does stress damage the brain? Biol Psychiatry 45:797–805, 1999b

Chu K, Kang DW, Kim HJ, et al: Diffusion-weighted imaging abnormalities in Wernicke encephalopathy: reversible cytotoxic edema? Arch Neurol 59:123–127, 2002

Csernansky JG: Structural MRI as a tool for the study of neurotoxicity and neurodegenerative disorders. J Anal Toxicol 25:414–418, 2001

Gilman S: Imaging the brain. N Engl J Med 338:812–819, 1998

Gurvits TV, Shenton ME, Hokama H, et al: Magnetic resonance imaging study of hippocampal volume in chronic combat-related post-traumatic stress disorder. Biol Psychiatry 40:1091–1099, 1996

Jones DK, Dardis R, Ervine M, et al: Cluster analysis of diffusion tensor magnetic resonance images in human head injury. Neurosurgery 47:306–313; discussion 313–314, 2000

Kotria KJ, Weinberger DR: Brain imaging in schizophrenia. Annu Rev Med 46:113–122, 1995

Loevner LA: Brain Imaging. St. Louis, MO, CV Mosby, 1999

Mann K, Mundle G, Strayle M, et al: Neuroimaging in alcoholism: CT and MRI results and clinical correlates. J Neural Transm Gen Sect 99(1–3):145–155, 1995

McCarley RW, Wible CG, Frumin M, et al: MRI anatomy of schizophrenia. Biol Psychiatry 45:1099–1119, 1999

McConnell HW, Snyder PJ (eds): Psychiatric Comorbidity in Epilepsy. Washington, DC, American Psychiatric Press, 1998

Nair TR, Christensen JD, Kingsbury SJ, et al: Progression of cerebroventricular enlargement and the subtyping of schizophrenia. Psychiatry Res 74:141–150, 1997

Narayn M, Bremner JD, Kumar A: Neuroanatomic substrates of late-life mental disorders. J Geriatr Psychiatry Neurol 12:95–106, 1999

Pfefferbaum A, Marsh L: Structural brain imaging in schizophrenia. Clin Neurosci 3:105–111, 1995

Pinner G, Johnson H, Bouman WP, et al: Psychiatric manifestations of normal-pressure hydrocephalus. Int Psychogeriatr 9:465–470, 1997

Pitman RK, Shin LM, Rauch SL: Investigating the pathogenesis of posttraumatic stress disorder with neuroimaging. J Clin Psychiatry 62 (suppl 17):47–62, 2001

Price BH: Neurology's interface with psychiatry, in Hospitalist Neurology (Blue Books of Practical Neurology, Vol 19). Edited by Samuels MA. Boston, MA, Butterworth-Heinemann Medical, 1999, pp 619–649

Sheline Y: Neuroanatomical changes associated with unipolar major depression. Neuroscientist 4:331–334, 1998

Stewart R: Neuroimaging in dementia and depression. Curr Opin Psychiatry 14(4):371–375, 2001

Ward PB: Structural brain imaging and the prevention of schizophrenia: can we identify neuroanatomical markers for young people at risk for the development of schizophrenia? Aust N Z J Psychiatry 34:S127–S130, 2000

Yock H: Magnetic Resonance Imaging of the Central Nervous System: A Teaching File. St. Louis, MO, Elsevier, 2001

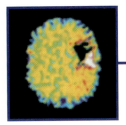

3

Positron Emission Tomography and Single Photon Emission Computed Tomography

Darin D. Dougherty, M.D., M.Sc.
Scott L. Rauch, M.D.
Alan J. Fischman, M.D., Ph.D.

Whereas computed tomography (CT; see Chapter 1 in this volume) and magnetic resonance imaging (MRI; see Chapter 2 in this volume) provide structural images of the brain, positron emission tomography (PET) and single photon emission computed tomography (SPECT) are radiological technologies that are used to measure numerous aspects of brain function. PET and SPECT, along with functional magnetic resonance imaging (fMRI; see Chapter 4 in this volume), are powerful tools for neuroscience research. Although PET and SPECT are still primarily research tools in the field of psychiatry, there is growing clinical utility for these methodologies. We begin this chapter by briefly describing the principles that underlie these methods. We

then discuss the use of PET and SPECT in both the clinical psychiatry and neuroscience research environments. Finally, we propose future directions for the use of PET and SPECT in psychiatry.

Principles of PET and SPECT

Positron Emission Tomography

Positron Emission

PET measures radioactive decay in order to form images of biological tissue function. Specifically, unstable nuclides are introduced into the organism being studied, and the PET camera detects the resulting radioactive decay and uses these data to construct functional images. Commonly used positron-emitting nuclides in PET studies include 11-carbon (^{11}C), 15-oxygen (^{15}O), 18-fluorine (^{18}F), and 13-nitrogen (^{13}N) (Table 3–1). These nuclides are incorporated into the desired molecules, resulting in a radiopharmaceutical (see subsection titled "Radiopharmaceuticals" later in this chapter). Because carbon, oxygen, hydrogen (18-fluorine is substituted for an existing hydrogen atom), and nitrogen constitute the building blocks of all organic molecules, their nuclides are particularly useful in radiopharmaceuticals designed to study biological processes.

Table 3–1. Radionuclides used in PET studies

Radionuclide	Half-life (minutes)	Common forms
^{15}Oxygen	2.0	$C^{15}O_2$, $H_2^{15}O_2$
^{13}Nitrogen	10.0	$^{13}NH_3$
^{11}Carbon	20.4	$^{11}CO_2$, ^{11}CO, $^{11}CH_3$
^{18}Fluorine	110.0	$^{18}F_2$, $H^{18}F$

Note. PET=positron emission tomography.

Because these unstable nuclides possess an excess of protons, they emit a *positron* (a positively charged atomic particle) in order to return to a more stable state. Soon after being emitted from the atom, the positively charged positron collides with a negatively charged *electron*. This collision results in an *annihilation event* wherein the mass of these particles is converted to energy in the form of two gamma photons, which travel in exactly opposite (180 degrees) directions from one another. The PET camera is designed to measure these gamma photons, or *gamma rays.*

Camera

To best detect the gamma rays resulting from the positron–electron annihilation event, the PET camera is designed as a series of *scintillation detectors* arrayed in a ringlike fashion. These scintillation detectors are crystalline and convert energy from gamma rays into light. Behind the scintillation detectors are *photomultiplier tubes,* which convert this light into data that are sent to the computer associated with the PET camera. The biological tissue being studied (be it the head or thorax of a human or an animal) is placed inside this ring, a radiopharmaceutical is introduced into the organism (usually intravenously), the radiopharmaceutical is redistributed in tissue according to the properties of the radiopharmaceutical, and the resulting gamma-ray emission is measured. Opposing detectors in the ring are coupled to form a *coincidence circuit* (Figure 3–1). Because the gamma rays from an annihilation event project exactly 180 degrees from each other, when gamma rays strike opposing detectors it is presumed that the annihilation event occurred at some point along the line

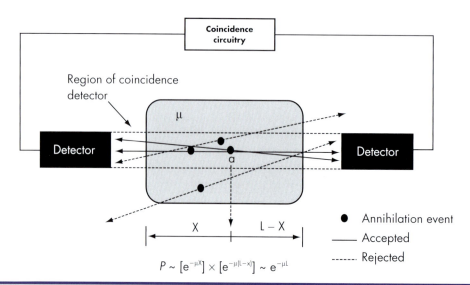

$$P \sim [e^{-\mu X}] \times [e^{-\mu(L-x)}] \sim e^{-\mu L}$$

Figure 3–1. Basic principles of annihilation–coincidence detection.
For an event to be recorded, both photons must arrive at the detectors within the resolving time of the coincidence circuitry. Events registered by only a single detector are rejected—"electronic collimation."
Source. Reprinted from Fischman AJ, Alpert NM, Babich JW, et al.: "The Role of Positron Emission Tomography in Pharmacokinetic Analysis." *Drug Metabolism Review* 29(4):923–956, 1997. Copyright 1997, Marcel Dekker, Inc. Used with permission.

connecting the two detectors. Sophisticated computer algorithms (a description of which is beyond the scope of this chapter) are then used to convert the data from all of these coincidence events into tomographic (cross-sectional) images of the tissue in question. The images produced by today's PET cameras have a maximum spatial resolution of approximately 3–5 millimeters (mm).

Single Photon Emission Computed Tomography

Photon Emission

SPECT differs from PET in that the radioactive process measured by SPECT does not result from a positron–electron collision. Instead, SPECT nuclides capture orbiting electrons in order to return to a more stable state. These single photons travel in just one direction, unlike the dual photons in PET nuclides, which travel in opposite directions (for this reason, PET is sometimes referred to as *dual photon* emission computed tomography). Commonly used SPECT nuclides include 99m-technetium (^{99m}Tc) and 123-iodine (^{123}I) (Table 3–2). These nuclides can often be incorporated in biological molecules of interest, although they are not as versatile as PET nuclides. The SPECT camera is designed to detect the emission of single photons from these nuclides.

Camera

Because SPECT nuclides produce a single photon, coincidence circuits like those employed by PET are not

Table 3–2. Radionuclides used in SPECT studies

Radionuclide	Half-life
^{99m}Technetium	6.0 hours
^{123}Iodine	13.0 hours
^{133}Xenon	5.3 days

Note. SPECT=single photon emission computed tomography.

useful. Instead, *collimators* are overlaid onto the radiation detectors that comprise the SPECT camera (Figure 3–2). The collimators are generally made of lead and contain thousands of small holes. These holes have a small diameter so that only photons that are traveling in a relatively parallel trajectory may pass through to the detector. The data that do reach the radiation detectors are constructed into an image by means of tomographic techniques similar to those used for PET studies. Many photons are deflected or filtered out and thus do not reach the detector, and it is this circumstance that is responsible for the limited sensitivity of SPECT.

Radiopharmaceuticals

In essence, a radiopharmaceutical is any molecule involved in a biological process of interest that can be effectively coupled with a radionuclide. For example, H_2O or CO_2 can be labeled with ^{15}O to be used as a marker of blood flow, fluorodeoxyglucose can be la-

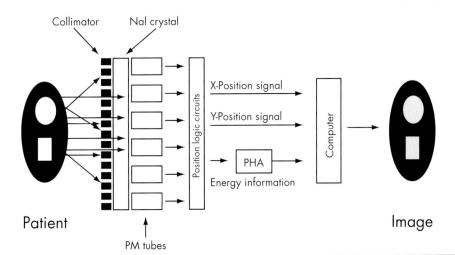

Figure 3–2. Basic components of a single-photon imaging system.
NaI=sodium iodide; PM=photomultiplier; PHA=pulse height analyzer.
Source. Reprinted from Fischman AJ, Alpert NM, Babich JW, et al.: "The Role of Positron Emission Tomography in Pharmacokinetic Analysis." *Drug Metabolism Review* 29(4):923–956, 1997. Copyright 1997, Marcel Dekker, Inc. Used with permission.

beled with ^{18}F to measure glucose metabolism, and a number of radionuclides can be used in the synthesis of radiopharmaceuticals that bind to different neuroreceptors. Both PET and SPECT studies can be used to study dynamic processes by sequential imaging following the introduction of the radiopharmaceutical of interest. Characterization of the regional uptake and washout of the radiopharmaceutical over time allows for quantification of blood flow, glucose metabolism, or neuroreceptor binding.

A number of important factors must be considered in the development of a radiopharmaceutical. First, the coupling of a radionuclide with a biological molecule of interest to form a radiopharmaceutical should not modify the biological or biochemical properties of the molecule of interest in any way. Second, for receptor studies, the radiopharmaceutical should have a high affinity for the target process. For example, if the radiopharmaceutical is designed to characterize serotonin type 2 (5-hydroxytryptamine$_2$ [5-HT$_2$]) receptors, it should have a high affinity for 5-HT$_2$ receptors. Third, the radiopharmaceutical's affinity for the target process should be much greater than its affinity for other biological processes (e.g., a radiopharmaceutical designed to characterize 5-HT$_2$ receptors must have much lower dopamine receptor affinity than 5-HT$_2$ receptor affinity). In other words, the radiopharmaceutical should be highly selective for the target. Fourth, a useful radiopharmaceutical generally must clear from nonspecific binding sites and the blood in a timely manner. This property is vitally important for optimizing target-to-background ratios. Fifth, as the radiopharmaceutical is metabolized, it is important that the metabolites be pharmacologically inactive. Active metabolites that bind to the site of interest represent a significant confound. Sixth, the radiopharmaceutical should be sufficiently lipophilic to be able to readily cross the blood–brain barrier. Seventh, the dose of the radiopharmaceutical administered for a PET or SPECT study should have no physiological activity. Because PET and SPECT are so exquisitely sensitive (i.e., capable of detecting radiopharmaceuticals at concentrations as low as 10^{-12} moles), the doses typically administered for a PET or SPECT study (often referred to as a "tracer dose") are rarely physiologically active. Thus, even molecules such as cocaine are routinely labeled with a nuclide and used as a radiopharmaceutical in human PET and SPECT studies at a concentration that has no physiological effects. Finally, rapidity of synthesis of the radiopharmaceutical is important, because the radionuclide is decaying even as it is being coupled with the molecule of interest.

Data Analysis

Information resulting from PET and SPECT studies may be examined at a number of levels. The simplest level is qualitative, in which the resulting images are visually inspected. This approach is used in clinical studies (e.g., glucose metabolism study for possible central nervous system neoplasm) and is sufficient for these applications. If quantitative information is desired (typically for research purposes), there are two ways of analyzing PET or SPECT data.

The simplest quantitative method involves calculating the ratio of the radiopharmaceutical's uptake in regions of interest to its uptake in reference regions. For example, if one conducted a PET or SPECT study with a radiopharmaceutical designed to bind to dopamine receptors, this reference method could be used to calculate the ratio of uptake in the striatum (rich in dopamine receptors) to uptake in the cerebellum (few dopamine receptors). Alternatively, some studies calculate the ratio of glucose metabolism in a region of interest to global (or whole-brain) glucose metabolism.

The more sophisticated method of quantitatively analyzing PET or SPECT data involves more complex mathematical procedures. It is beyond the scope of this chapter to describe these procedures in detail; suffice it to say that different mathematical procedures are used to calculate variables that represent various aspects of the biological process of interest. For example, blood flow or glucose metabolism can be ascertained throughout the brain at the level of resolution of the PET or SPECT camera. If these data are collected during two different states (e.g., at rest and during a cognitive task), changes in blood flow or glucose metabolism can be assessed statistically on a voxel-by-voxel basis (a voxel is the three-dimensional equivalent of a pixel). Another example of a mathematical process used for quantitatively assessing PET or SPECT data is kinetic modeling for neuroreceptor studies. Kinetic modeling assumes that the radiopharmaceutical is present in a number of states, or *compartments*. Such compartments may include plasma, free in tissue, specifically bound in tissue, nonspecifically bound in tissue, and so forth. The appropriate number of compartments may vary from radiopharmaceutical to radiopharmaceutical, given that the best model depends on the physiological properties of the radiopharmaceutical in question (e.g., reversible binding versus irreversible binding, bolus injection of radiopharmaceutical versus continuous infusion). *Rate constants* are variables that represent the rate of movement of the radiopharmaceutical from one compartment to another. Values for some rate constants are provided by the PET or SPECT data and concurrent blood sampling. Once these values are available, mathematical modeling allows for estimation of the other values. This kinetic modeling may then yield estimations of receptor binding, including binding affinity (K_d), receptor occupancy (B_{max}), and binding potential (the ratio of B_{max} to K_d).

What Can PET and SPECT Measure?

PET can measure both blood flow and glucose metabolism as indices of neuronal activity. Typically, ^{15}O compounds (which have a short half-life—approximately 2 minutes) are used to measure blood flow. These ^{15}O compounds may be injected ($H_2^{15}O$) or inhaled ($C^{15}O_2$). Alternatively, ^{18}F-fluorodeoxyglucose (FDG) is used to measure glucose metabolism. In short, ^{18}F-FDG is phosphorylated by the brain through the same pathway as glucose. However, ^{18}F-FDG is unable to continue beyond this point in the metabolic pathway and is trapped in neurons. This trapping of ^{18}F-FDG, often referred to as ^{18}F-FDG uptake, serves as a marker of metabolic activity.

Whereas PET can measure both blood flow and glucose metabolism as indices of neuronal activity, SPECT can measure only blood flow. A number of ^{99m}Tc- and ^{123}I-labeled compounds—including ^{99m}Tc-hexamethylpropyleneamine oxime (HMPAO), ^{99m}Tc-ethylene cysteinate dimer (ECD), and ^{123}I-isopropyliodoamphetamine (IMP)—may be used for SPECT blood flow studies. The ^{99m}Tc-labeled radiopharmaceuticals are predominantly used for such SPECT studies, because they demonstrate superior pharmacokinetics and are less costly to synthesize in comparison with the other SPECT radiopharmaceuticals available for this purpose.

Both PET and SPECT are able to use a number of radiopharmaceuticals to measure different aspects of neurotransmitter function (Table 3–3). Different radiopharmaceuticals are capable of quantitating neurotransmitter synthesis and of characterizing pre- and postsynaptic neurotransmitter receptors as well as neurotransmitter transporters or reuptake sites. In addition, exciting new research has led to the development of experimental radiopharmaceuticals designed to study ever more complex biological processes, including protein synthesis, second-messenger systems, DNA replication, and gene expression.

Clinical Applications

Dementia

There are numerous causes of the symptoms of dementia. The most common cause of dementia in the

Table 3–3. Radiopharmaceuticals used in PET and SPECT studies

Radiopharmaceutical	Target
PET	
$C^{15}O_2$, $H_2^{15}O$	Blood flow
^{18}F-fluorodeoxyglucose	Glucose metabolism
^{11}C-SCH-23390	D_1
^{11}C-raclopride	D_2
^{11}C-altropane	Dopamine transporter
^{18}F-setoperone	$5\text{-}HT_2$
^{11}C-WAY-100635	$5\text{-}HT_{1A}$
^{11}C-flumazenil	Benzodiazepine
^{11}C-carfentanyl	μ opioid
^{11}C-diprenorphine	Nonselective opioid
SPECT	
^{99m}Tc-HMPAO	Blood flow
^{99m}Tc-ECD	Blood flow
^{133}Xe	Blood flow
^{133}I-β-CIT	Dopamine transporter/ serotonin transporter
^{133}I-altropane	Dopamine transporter
^{133}I-epidipride	D_2
^{133}I-IBZM	D_2

Note. 5-HT = 5-hydroxytryptamine (serotonin); D = dopamine; HMPAO = hexamethylpropyleneamine oxime; ECD = ethylene cysteinate dimer; IBZM = iodobenzamide; PET = positron emission tomography; SPECT = single photon emission computed tomography.

United States is Alzheimer's disease. Although diagnosis of Alzheimer's disease can often be made after a clinical and neuropsychological evaluation, continued diagnostic uncertainty is not uncommon even after a thorough evaluation. Any tool that can increase the sensitivity and specificity of diagnosis would be tremendously valuable. This is especially the case in view of the fact that effective treatments for Alzheimer's disease are becoming available. A growing body of literature suggests that PET and SPECT are useful tools for assessing patients with possible Alzheimer's disease. Studies have demonstrated that PET and SPECT have high sensitivity and specificity in diagnosing Alzheimer's disease and can also play an important role in differentiating Alzheimer's disease from other causes of dementia.

PET studies of subjects with suspected Alzheimer's disease almost exclusively use ^{18}F-FDG; SPECT studies typically use the ^{99m}Tc-labeled radiopharmaceuticals HMPAO and ECD. The classic pattern (Figure 3–3) seen in PET and SPECT studies of patients with Alzheimer's disease is bilateral (often symmetrical) hypoperfusion or hypometabolism in the parietal and temporal cortices with sparing of the somatosensory and

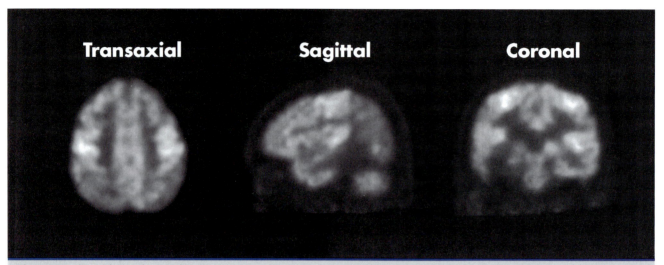

Figure 3–3. Fluorodeoxyglucose positron emission tomography (FDG PET) images of a patient with Alzheimer's disease.
Note that metabolism is decreased in all cortical regions except the somatosensory cortex. This preservation of the somatosensory cortex is sometimes referred to as the "ear-muff sign."

visual cortices. As the disease progresses in severity, the deficits detectable on functional imaging spread anteriorly to include the frontal cortex. Changes visible on PET and SPECT images occur well before structural changes are visible with CT or MRI. Many other forms of dementia have characteristic patterns of hypoperfusion or hypometabolism detectable by PET or SPECT that can aid in their differentiation from Alzheimer's disease. Although the total number of causes of dementia is too large to allow for a complete listing of PET and SPECT findings for each cause, some representative examples may help elucidate how PET and SPECT can aid in the differential diagnosis of dementia. PET or SPECT studies of patients with Pick's disease usually demonstrate hypoperfusion or hypometabolism that is exclusive to frontal regions of the brain, with posterior regions spared. Patients with multi-infarct dementia typically demonstrate patchy areas of hypoperfusion or hypometabolism that correspond to lesions seen with structural imaging. Many other types of dementia exist, including human immunodeficiency virus (HIV) dementia, Lewy body disease, Lyme encephalopathy, and Creutzfeldt-Jakob disease; PET and SPECT findings for these and other causes of dementia are relatively nonspecific and may include global hypoperfusion or hypometabolism as well as diffuse regions demonstrating functional deficits.

The use of PET and SPECT for the evaluation of dementia has been studied with increasing rigor in recent years. A recent study conducted by Silverman et al. (2001) examined ^{18}F-FDG PET data from 284 patients being evaluated for dementia. Longitudinal follow-up consisted of either a minimum of 2 years of clinical follow-up after the PET study or postmortem histopathological diagnosis. This large study demonstrated that PET was capable of detecting Alzheimer's disease with a sensitivity of 94% and a specificity of 73%. In addition, the authors concluded that normal PET scan results in this population indicated that progression of cognitive impairment was unlikely to occur during the follow-up period. Other studies examining the relationship between PET ^{18}F-FDG findings and apolipoprotein E-4 allele status (presence of the allele is a known genetic risk factor for developing Alzheimer's disease) have demonstrated that even a single copy of the allele in persons without dementia (with or without a familial risk for Alzheimer's disease) is associated with hypometabolism in parietal and temporal cortices (Reiman et al. 2001). Combining PET or SPECT imaging with genotyping may eventually prove to be an effective means of detecting preclinical Alzheimer's disease. Finally, studies focusing on new PET radiopharmaceuticals specifically designed to bind to the beta-amyloid plaques that are histologically pathognomonic for Alzheimer's disease show particular promise for early detection of Alzheimer's disease (Petrella et al. 2003).

Epilepsy

The diagnosis of epilepsy is usually based on clinical symptoms and the results of electroencephalogram

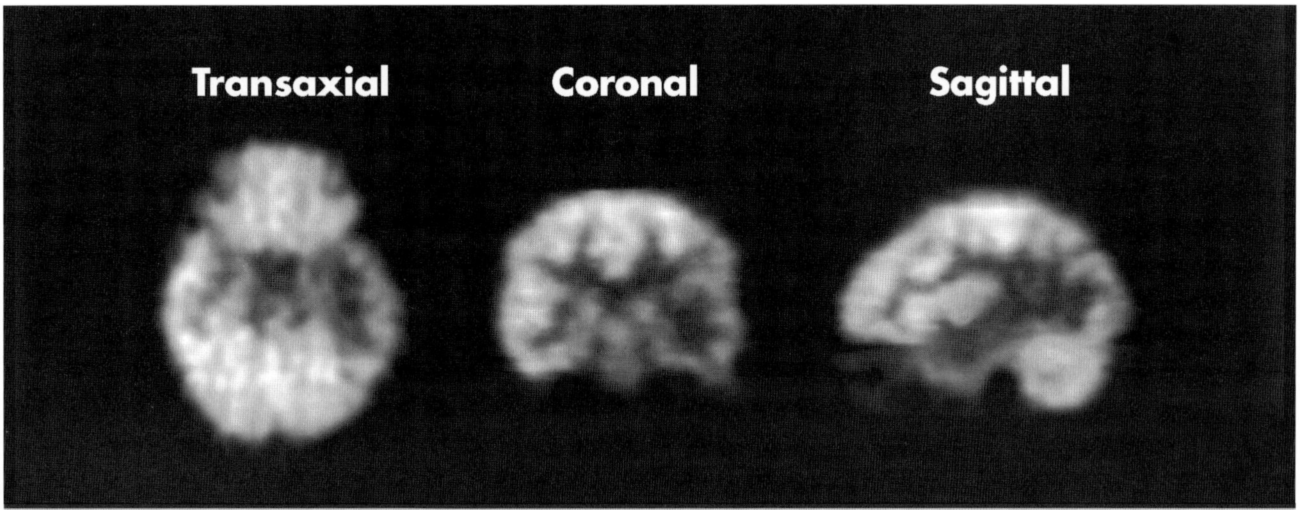

Figure 3–4. Fluorodeoxyglucose positron emission tomography (FDG PET) images of a patient with temporal lobe epilepsy.
These images were acquired during an interictal period. Note that metabolism is decreased in the brain region that contains the seizure focus, compared with the rest of the cortex. If FDG PET images were acquired during the ictal period, metabolism would be increased in the same region.

(EEG) studies. At times, however, EEG studies demonstrate no abnormalities despite the presence of clinical symptoms consistent with seizures. In these instances, PET or SPECT imaging can be indispensable in confirming the diagnosis of epilepsy. Characteristic findings include hyperperfusion or hypermetabolism at the seizure locus during a seizure and hypoperfusion or hypometabolism at the seizure locus during the interictal period (Figure 3–4). An important role of PET or SPECT in the management of epilepsy is in the localization of a seizure locus prior to surgical resection for treatment-refractory cases.

Cerebrovascular Disease

As has already been described, both PET and SPECT are able to measure blood flow. Thus, it logically follows that these modalities could be useful for the diagnosis and assessment of cerebrovascular disease. The most promising use of perfusion PET and/or SPECT studies in cerebrovascular disease is for the evaluation of acute ischemia. SPECT cameras and the ^{99m}Tc-labeled SPECT radiopharmaceuticals are more widely available than PET cameras and ^{15}O-labeled compounds. Thus, although both modalities are effective for the evaluation of acute ischemia, SPECT is much more commonly used than PET.

SPECT perfusion studies allow for almost immediate detection of hypoperfusion after an acute ischemic event (Figure 3–5). By contrast, it may be many hours before structural changes following an acute ischemic event can be identified with CT, and these structural changes may never be seen during the acute phase if standard MRI is used. In addition, SPECT perfusion studies are able to detect hypoperfusion not only at the site of the vascular event but also in brain regions distant from the focal event. These remote regions of hypoperfusion often occur as a result of acute ischemia at a separate site. However, whereas the resulting necrotic damage at the site of the acute ischemia is often permanent, the hypoperfusion in remote brain regions may resolve over time. Nonetheless, during the acute ischemic event, the hypoperfusion in the remote brain regions may cause symptoms that are erroneously attributed to the focal event. By comparison, structural scans rarely demonstrate changes in regions distant from the focal event.

It is important to note that SPECT's sensitivity in detecting an acute ischemic event decreases as the stroke evolves, because the initial phase of hypoperfusion is followed by increased perfusion at the lesion site over the next 1–5 days. SPECT images of the site may appear normal during this interval until tissue at the site returns to a chronic, hypoperfused state; this may not occur for as long as 20–30 days after the event. New MRI techniques such as diffusion-weighted MRI (see Chapter 2 in this volume) may be as sensitive as PET or SPECT for the evaluation of acute ischemia. Diffusion-weighted MRI also has greater spatial resolu-

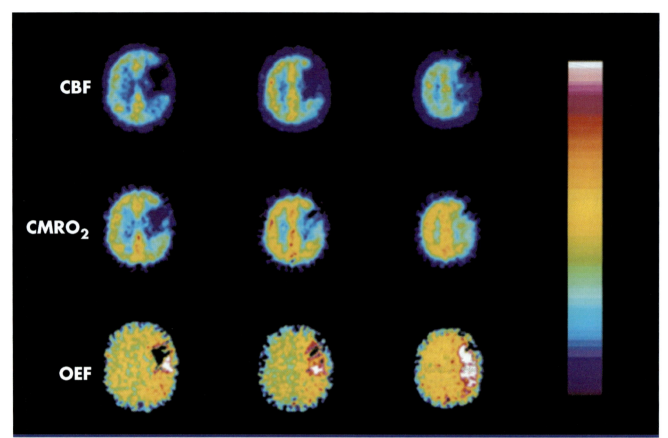

Figure 3–5. 15-Oxygen positron emission tomography (^{15}O PET) data acquired from a patient during an acute ischemic event.

^{15}O PET data can be used to measure a number of indices of neuronal activity. This image shows that cerebral blood flow (CBF), cerebral metabolic rate of oxygen (CMRO$_2$), and oxygen extraction fraction (OEF) are all markedly decreased at the site of the acute ischemic event.

tion than PET or SPECT and is more widely available. Studies comparing the sensitivity and specificity of diffusion-weighted MRI with those of PET and/or SPECT for the evaluation of acute ischemia are currently in progress. Finally, it is worth mentioning that studies assessing the utility of PET and/or SPECT in the evaluation of other cerebrovascular diseases, such as transient ischemic attacks and subarachnoid hemorrhage, are under way.

Head Trauma

CT and MRI are the studies of choice for evaluation of acute head trauma. Some studies have demonstrated that the degree of abnormality detected by PET or SPECT following head trauma correlates with prognosis. Notwithstanding, PET and SPECT studies are rarely performed after acute head trauma. PET and SPECT studies may be more useful than structural imaging modalities during the chronic phase after head

trauma, given that they are better able to detect subtle abnormalities. This increased sensitivity of PET and SPECT may be especially valuable in cases where structural scans yield normal findings but cognitive or affective disturbances are present. Abnormal PET or SPECT findings in these cases not only are diagnostically useful but also may play an important role in the planning and monitoring of rehabilitation therapy. In fact, studies have demonstrated that abnormalities on neuropsychological testing correlate with deficits found on functional imaging in head trauma patients and that improvements in testing results correlate with increased brain perfusion in these patients.

Cerebral Neoplasms

Neoplastic lesions, whether they are primary or metastatic, typically have greater metabolic demands than surrounding tissue. This increased metabolic demand allows for successful imaging of neoplasms

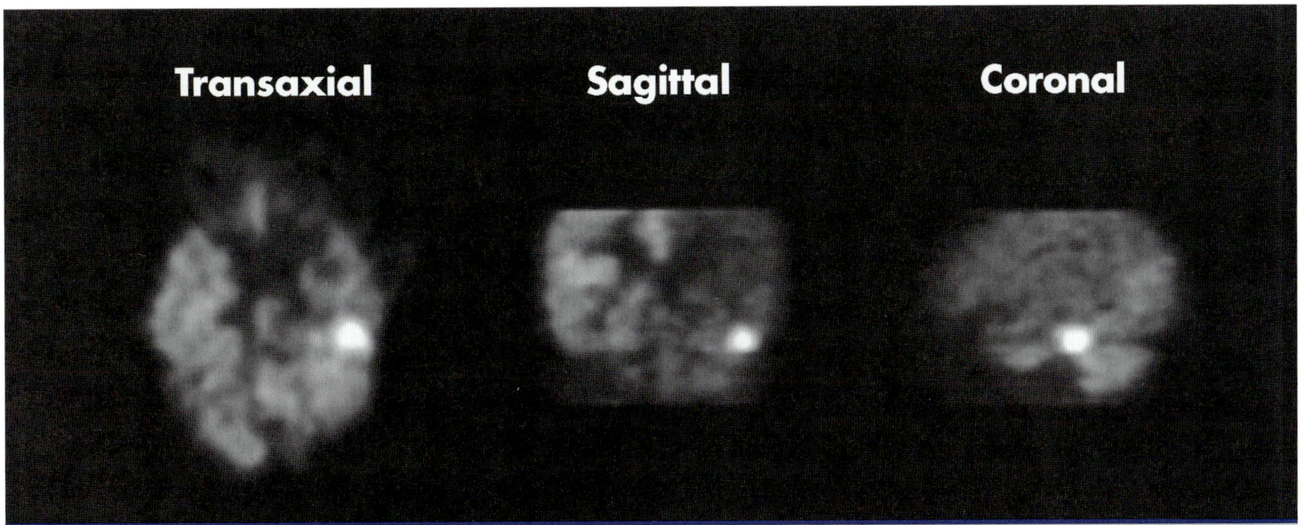

Figure 3–6. Fluorodeoxyglucose positron emission tomography (FDG PET) images of a patient with a neoplasm. As these images demonstrate, neoplasms are typically hypermetabolic in comparison with healthy brain tissue.

with PET and SPECT. The state-of-the-art functional imaging modality for detecting neoplasms is ^{18}F-FDG PET. As a result of the increased glucose metabolism of the neoplasms, the lesions appear hypermetabolic on PET images (Figure 3–6). SPECT radiopharmaceuticals that are effective for detecting neoplasms including ^{201}Tl-thallous chloride and ^{99m}Tc-sestamibi.

Parkinson's Disease

Parkinson's disease is caused by degeneration of dopaminergic neurons in the substantia nigra, leading to decreased dopamine in the striatum. As many as 75% of dopaminergic neurons in the substantia nigra may be destroyed before patients begin to demonstrate symptoms. Current studies are examining whether PET and SPECT may play a role in diagnosing Parkinson's disease not only in patients with symptoms but also in susceptible individuals before the onset of symptoms. Two avenues of research show promise: radiopharmaceuticals designed to measure presynaptic dopamine synthesis (e.g., ^{18}F-DOPA for PET) and radiopharmaceuticals designed to measure dopamine transporter binding (e.g., ^{123}I-beta-CIT and ^{131}I-altropane for SPECT, ^{11}C-altropane and ^{11}C-CFT for PET). Both of these components of the dopaminergic system serve as neuronal markers for determining the degree of loss of dopaminergic presynaptic terminals in the striatum. A number of studies have demonstrated decreased binding of these radiopharmaceuticals in the striatum of patients with Parkinson's disease (Figure

3–7). Whereas traditional pharmacotherapies for Parkinson's disease have focused on increasing dopaminergic tone in the striatum, newer agents designed to halt or even reverse neurodegeneration are currently being developed. PET and SPECT could play an important role in serially evaluating patients' response to these newer agents.

Research Applications
Functional Neuroanatomy

PET and SPECT studies of regional cerebral blood flow (rCBF) and regional cerebral metabolic rate (rCMR) are commonly used in functional neuroanatomy studies. fMRI is another important tool in this area of research (see Chapter 4 in this volume). There are a number of different paradigms that can be used for studying brain function in both patient populations and healthy volunteers.

The simplest type of functional neuroanatomy investigation is the resting-state study, in which subjects simply undergo PET or SPECT imaging while at rest (this nominal resting state is often referred to as a *neutral state*). Typically, subjects are injected with ^{18}F-FDG for PET or ^{99m}Tc-HMPAO or ^{99m}Tc-ECD for SPECT in a quiet room with as little stimulation as possible. After enough time has elapsed for complete uptake of the radiopharmaceutical to occur, subjects are placed within the PET or SPECT camera, and data are acquired. Neutral-state studies are useful for comparing

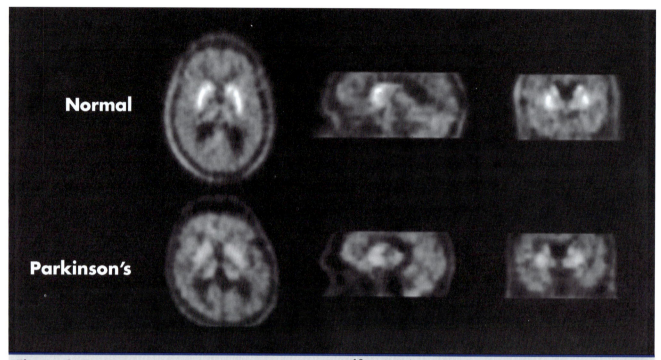

Figure 3–7.   Positron emission tomography studies with ¹⁸F-DOPA, a radiopharmaceutical used to measure presynaptic dopamine synthesis.
The degree of binding of this radiopharmaceutical in the striatum is a marker for the number of intact dopaminergic neurons in this brain region. As these images indicate, there is far less binding of ¹⁸F-DOPA in the striatum of the patient with Parkinson's disease in comparison with the healthy volunteer.

resting rCBF or rCMR across populations. To date, these studies have been used only in research applications, given that differences across populations are usually not detectable in an individual scan; rather, pooling of subjects is required. Neutral-state studies have demonstrated that groups of patients with major depression show decreased rCBF or rCMR in frontal regions compared with control populations (Figure 3–8) and that groups of patients with obsessive-compulsive disorder demonstrate increased rCBF or rCMR in orbitofrontal cortex and the head of the caudate nucleus.

Although neutral-state studies have provided a great deal of valuable information regarding the pathophysiology of numerous psychiatric illnesses, studies that assess brain function during specific tasks may be a more powerful tool. Just as electrocardiogram data collected during a cardiac stress test may uncover cardiac abnormalities not detectable with a resting electrocardiogram, functional neuroimaging studies that use activation paradigms may be more sensitive than neutral-state studies. Of course, these studies may be conducted in patient populations and in healthy volunteers. SPECT is not as useful for these activation studies as PET or fMRI (see Chapter 4 in this volume

for a more detailed description of fMRI), because generally only one image can be collected per day with SPECT. By comparison, the use of ¹⁵O-labeled radiopharmaceuticals with PET permits investigators to conduct numerous studies in a single day. Because the half-life of ¹⁵O is approximately 2 minutes, all radioactivity dissipates within approximately 10 minutes (5 half-lives) and another study may then be performed. Therefore, as many as 12 separate ¹⁵O PET studies may be conducted in a single individual within a few hours. Subjects are asked to perform various tasks, including activation and baseline tasks, during separate studies. For example, subjects may be instructed to follow a moving target with their eyes during one study, to watch a fixed target during another study, and to close their eyes during yet another study. By pooling data across subjects and then subtracting the baseline studies from the activation studies, investigators can determine which brain regions are involved in mediating the activation task (Figure 3–9). Again, as an example, if the closed-eye studies described earlier are subtracted from the fixed-target studies, the difference should reflect which brain regions are involved in looking at a fixed target. The number of activation tasks that can be employed in such studies is limitless;

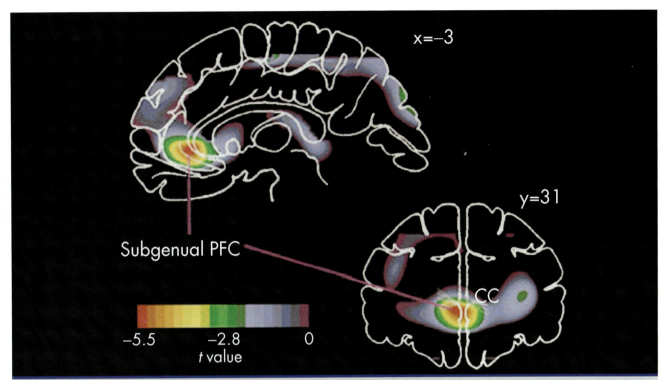

Figure 3–8. Coronal and sagittal sections showing a region of decreased glucose metabolism in depressed patients relative to control subjects.

CC = corpus callosum; PFC = prefrontal cortex.

Source. Reprinted from Drevets WC, Price JL, Simpson JR Jr, et al.: "Subgenual Prefrontal Cortex Abnormalities in Mood Disorders." *Nature* 386:824–827, 1997. Copyright 1997, Macmillan Publishers Ltd. Used by permission from *Nature* (www.nature.com/nature).

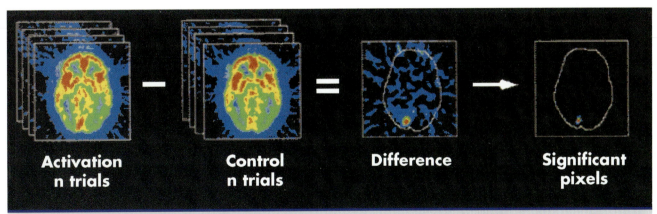

Figure 3–9. Illustration of the methodology for positron emission tomography (PET) activation studies using blood flow tracers.

A series of scans are acquired in activated and control states and are subtracted to produce a difference image. A statistical test is applied to the data to determine which changes in the difference image are statistically significant. This example shows the robust response to a hemifield stimulation of the visual system with a reversing checkerboard pattern in a PET study that used $[H_2{}^{15}O]$ as the tracer. The activated area in the visual cortex can be clearly seen.

Source. Reprinted from Cherry SR, Phelps ME: "Imaging Brain Function With Positron Emission Tomography," in *Brain Mapping: The Methods.* Edited by Toga AW, Mazziotta JC. San Diego, CA, Academic Press, 1998. Copyright 1998, Elsevier Science Inc. (www.elsevier.com). Used with permission.

such paradigms have included cognitive tasks (e.g., tests of memory), affective tasks (e.g., eliciting various emotions with pictures, film, or audiotape), symptom provocation studies (e.g., inducing panic attack symptoms), and symptom capture studies (e.g., analyzing data to compare profiles associated with the presence of a spontaneous event, such as auditory hallucinations or motor tics).

Finally, whereas the research paradigms described in this section have the potential to further our knowledge of the pathophysiology of psychiatric illnesses, functional neuroimaging can also be used to assess treatment. Such assessment can be accomplished in two ways. First, a baseline functional neuroimaging study

can be conducted before subjects begin treatment. This baseline functional neuroimaging study may consist of a single neutral-state study or a number of activation studies. After subjects have completed the treatment trial, an analysis can be performed to determine whether rCBF or rCMR in different brain regions correlates with treatment response. This may be done in a categorical manner or by using continuous variables. The categorical analysis simply consists of dividing the cohort into responders and nonresponders and then comparing the two groups of scans. The differences correspond to brain regions where increased or decreased rCBF or rCMR at baseline correlates with subsequent treatment response or nonresponse (Figure 3–10). In the

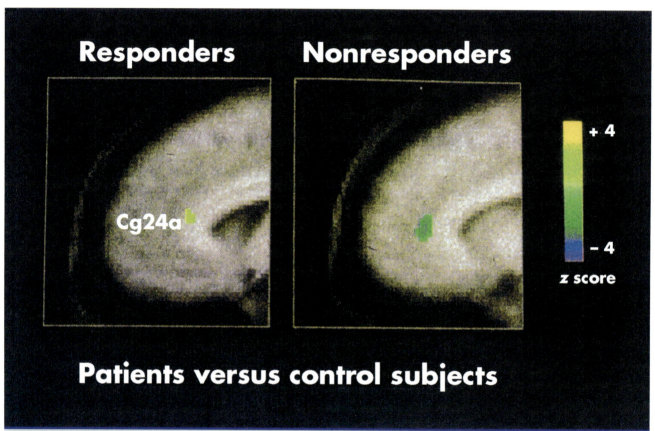

Figure 3–10. Categorical analysis of treatment response.
Shown are superimposed positron emission tomography scans and magnetic resonance images, sagittal view, from two groups of depressed patients compared with healthy control subjects. The z-score maps demonstrate differences in direction, magnitude, and extent of changes seen in rostral cingulate (Cg24a) glucose metabolism in patients versus control subjects. Cingulate hypometabolism (negative z values, shown in green) characterized the nonresponder group, whereas hypermetabolism (positive z values, shown in yellow) was seen in those who eventually responded to treatment.
Source. Reprinted from Mayberg HS, Brannan SK, Mahurin RK, et al.: "Cingulate Function in Depression: A Potential Predictor of Treatment Response." *Neuroreport* 8:1057–1061, 1997. Copyright 1997, Lippincott Williams & Wilkins (www.lww.com). Used with permission.

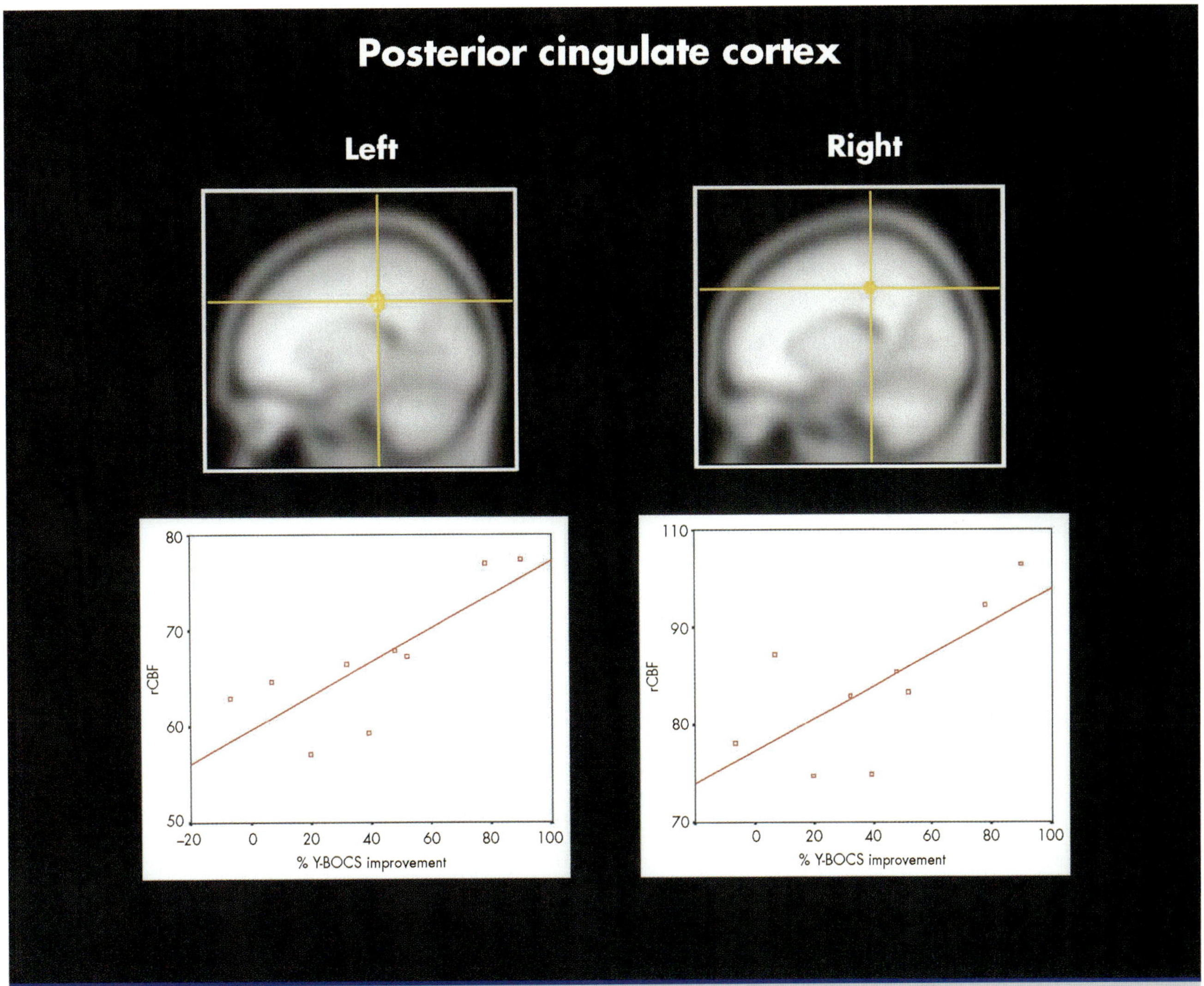

Posterior cingulate cortex

Left

Right

Figure 3–11.   Continuous-variable analysis of treatment response.
The upper panels show the locations of significant positive correlations between positron emission tomography measurements of regional cerebral blood flow (rCBF) in the posterior cingulate cortex bilaterally and subsequent fluvoxamine response as measured by percentage change in the Yale-Brown Obsessive Compulsive Scale (Y-BOCS) score, superimposed over the SPM99 (Statistical Parametric Mapping 99 [software program]) template in MNI (Montreal Neurological Institute) space for anatomic reference. The lower panels show the actual corresponding plots of percentage Y-BOCS improvement versus rCBF.
Source.   Reprinted from Rauch SL, Shin LM, Dougherty DD, et al.: "Predictors of Fluvoxamine Response in Contamination-Related Obsessive Compulsive Disorder: A PET Symptom Provocation Study." *Neuropsychopharmacology* 27:782–791, 2002. Copyright 2002, American College of Neuropsychopharmacology. Used by permission of Elsevier Science (www.elsevier.com).

continuous-variable analysis, all subjects are pooled together, and the degree of treatment response (e.g., percentage change in Beck Depression Inventory scores following treatment) is entered as a covariate for each individual study. This continuous-variable analysis reveals brain regions where baseline rCBF or rCMR positively or negatively correlates with subsequent treatment response (Figure 3–11). The second way to use functional neuroimaging to assess treatment is to collect PET or SPECT data both before and after treatment. All of the analyses described above can be conducted with the baseline data. However, the pooled pretreatment functional neuroimaging data can be compared with the posttreatment data to determine whether changes occur that may provide clues about the mechanism of action of the treatment being studied.

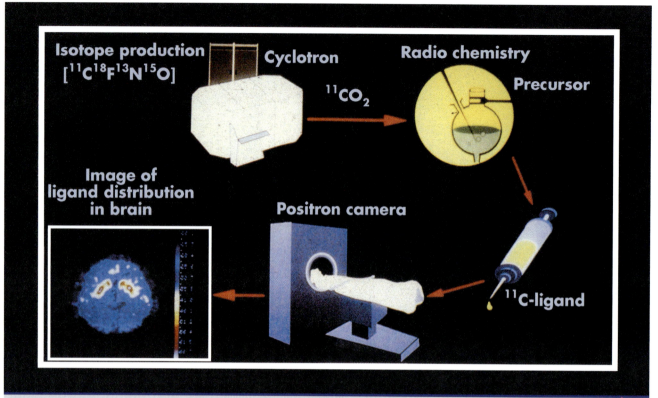

Figure 3–12. Schematic demonstrating steps involved in conducting a positron emission tomography study employing a radiopharmaceutical designed for neuroreceptor characterization.
Source. Reprinted from Sedvall G, Farde L, Persson A, et al.: "Imaging of Neurotransmitter Receptors in the Living Human Brain." *Archives of General Psychiatry* 43:995–1005, 1986. Copyright 1986, American Medical Association. Used with permission.

Neurochemistry

As described earlier, PET and SPECT can be used to characterize various aspects of neurotransmitter function (Figure 3–12). Table 3–3 presented a partial list of radiopharmaceuticals available for PET and SPECT studies and also indicated which aspect of neurotransmitter function each measures. If one views the results of a PET or SPECT neurochemistry study as equivalent to rCBF or rCMR data in the sense of paradigm design, it becomes evident that many of the studies described in the previous section could be conducted with neurochemistry data collected during PET or SPECT studies. For example, one could characterize 5-HT₂ receptors at rest in a population of patients with major depression and a population of healthy volunteers and compare the two groups; this would be equivalent to a neutral-state study.

Activation studies with PET or SPECT neurochemistry data can also be conducted. However, given the longer half-lives of ^{11}C and ^{18}F and the length of time required to conduct a single PET or SPECT neurochemistry study (approximately 90 minutes), generally only two such studies could be conducted on a single day. A baseline (resting or neutral state) PET or SPECT neurochemistry study is typically conducted first, followed by a second study identical to the first except that some type of perturbation is introduced during the second study. Examples include administration of a drug, assignment of a cognitive or affective activation task, or introduction of a form of external manipulation such as acupuncture. Thus, if 5-HT₂ receptor binding is determined first at rest and then during infusion of a drug, the two PET or SPECT studies can be compared with each another to determine the effect of the drug on 5-HT₂ binding. Along these same lines, PET or SPECT neurochemistry studies can be conducted before treatment or both before and after treatment, and all of the analyses employed in other functional neuroimaging studies designed to assess treatment can be used to analyze the PET or SPECT neurochemistry data.

Finally, PET and SPECT neurochemistry studies have the potential to play an important role in drug development, given that their methodologies are ideally suited for in vivo pharmacokinetic and pharmacodynamic studies. For example, a candidate molecule may be directly labeled with a radionuclide and injected into an animal or human subject as acquisition of PET or SPECT data is initiated (Figure 3–13). This allows the investigator to determine where in the brain the drug localizes, establish a dose-to-receptor occupancy curve, and assess the time course of clearance from the brain. The latter two pieces of information may be especially important for determining dose strength and dosing schedule. If the candidate molecule cannot be directly labeled with a radionuclide, an indirect method may be used (Figure 3–14). In this case, a baseline PET or SPECT study is performed with an existing radiopharmaceutical. The unlabeled drug is then administered,

following which another PET or SPECT study is conducted with the same radiopharmaceutical. For example, a candidate drug may be known to bind to 5-HT$_2$ receptors in vitro. A baseline PET study is performed with ^{18}F-setoperone, which is known to bind to 5-HT$_2$ receptors. Next, the PET study is repeated, but after administration of the unlabeled drug. The unlabeled drug will compete with ^{18}F-setoperone for the 5-HT$_2$ binding sites. The quantitative difference between the two studies in ^{18}F-setoperone binding as measured by the PET camera represents the degree of binding of the unlabeled drug to 5-HT$_2$ receptors.

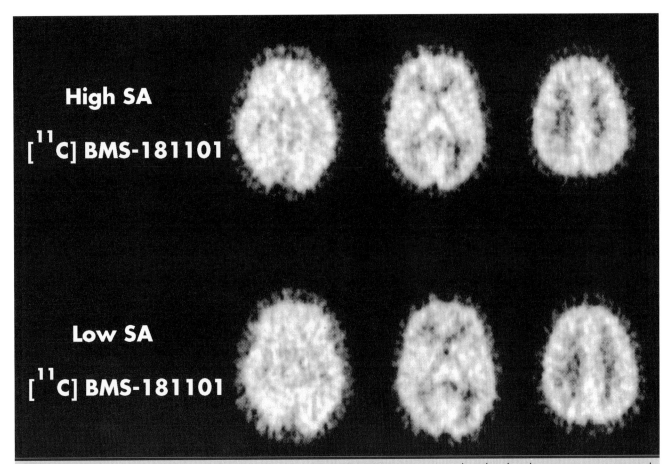

Figure 3–13. Direct method of drug evaluation: BMS-181101, a compound under development as a potential antidepressant, fails to demonstrate in vitro effects on serotonergic receptors.

A positron emission tomography study conducted to assess in vivo distribution of BMS-181101 in the central nervous system (CNS) used BMS-181101 labeled with the radionuclide ^{11}C. The images show the distribution of ^{11}C-BMS-181101 in the brain after high- *(top row)* and low- *(bottom row)* specific-activity (SA) injections. Note that there is no significant difference in the amount of specific binding between the high- and low-SA studies. These results indicate that the CNS distribution of ^{11}C-BMS-181101 is dominated by blood flow and that significant receptor-specific localization does not occur in any brain region. Further development of this drug was subsequently halted.

Source. Reprinted from Christian BT, Livni E, Babich JW, et al.: "Evaluation of Cerebral Pharmacokinetics of the Novel Antidepressant Drug, BMS-181101, by Positron Emission Tomography." *Journal of Pharmacology and Experimental Therapeutics* 279(1):325–331, 1996. Copyright 1996, American Society for Pharmacology and Experimental Therapeutics. Used with permission.

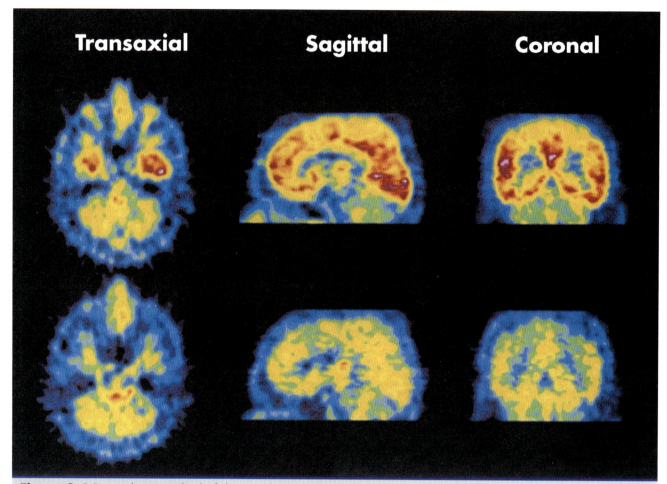

Transaxial   **Sagittal**   **Coronal**

Figure 3–14.   Indirect method of drug evaluation: Ziprasidone, a novel antipsychotic, shows a high affinity for serotonin 5-HT$_2$ receptors in vitro.

This study was conducted to determine the time course of 5-HT$_2$ receptor occupancy in healthy humans following a single oral dose of ziprasidone. Positron emission tomography (PET) studies with ^{18}F-setoperone, a radiopharmaceutical that selectively binds to 5-HT$_2$ receptors, were conducted in a group of healthy volunteers, first during a baseline state and then after a 40-mg dose of ziprasidone. Shown are transverse, sagittal, and coronal PET images of the brain of a healthy subject before *(upper row)* and 4 hours after *(lower row)* oral administration of 40 mg of ziprasidone. Note the marked decrease in ^{18}F-setoperone accumulation following dosing with ziprasidone, indicating displacement of ^{18}F-setoperone from 5-HT$_2$ binding sites.

Source.   Reprinted from Fischman AJ, Bonab AA, Babich JW, et al.: "Positron Emission Tomographic Analysis of Central 5-Hydroxytryptamine$_2$ Receptor Occupancy in Healthy Volunteers Treated With the Novel Antipsychotic Agent, Ziprasidone." *Journal of Pharmacology and Experimental Therapeutics* 279(3):939–947, 1996. Copyright 1996, American Society for Pharmacology and Experimental Therapeutics. Used with permission.

Future Directions

PET and SPECT technology has advanced considerably in recent decades. Although still used primarily for research in the psychiatric setting, PET and SPECT demonstrate growing promise for the clinical setting. Ongoing studies are examining the potential role of PET and SPECT in diagnosis and in predicting treatment response. As PET and SPECT technology continues to evolve, these potential clinical applications may come to fruition.

References/Suggested Readings

Cherry SR, Phelps ME: Imaging brain function with positron emission tomography, in Brain Mapping: The Methods. Edited by Toga AW, Mazziotta JC. San Diego, CA, Academic Press, 1996, pp 191–222

Dougherty DD, Rauch SL (eds): Psychiatric Neuroimaging Research: Contemporary Strategies. Washington, DC, American Psychiatric Publishing, 2001

Fischman AJ, Alpert NM, Babich JW, et al: The role of positron emission tomography in pharmacokinetic analysis. Drug Metabolism Review 29(4):923–956, 1997

Petrella JR, Coleman RE, Doraiswamy PM: Neuroimaging and early diagnosis of Alzheimer disease: a look to the future. Radiology 226:315–336, 2003

Reiman EM, Caselli RJ, Chen K, et al: Declining brain activity in cognitively normal apolipoprotein E epsilon 4 heterozygotes: a foundation for using positron emission tomography to efficiently test treatments to prevent Alzheimer's disease. Proc Natl Acad Sci U S A 98:3334–3339, 2001

Renshaw PF, Rauch SL: Neuroimaging in clinical psychiatry, in The Harvard Guide to Psychiatry, 3rd Edition. Edited by Nicholi AM Jr. Cambridge, MA, Belknap Press, 1999, pp 84–97

Silverman DH, Small GW, Chang CY, et al: Positron emission tomography in evaluation of dementia: regional brain metabolism and long-term outcome. JAMA 286:2120–2127, 2001

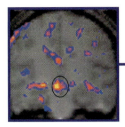

4

Functional Magnetic Resonance Imaging

Robert L. Savoy, Ph.D.
Randy L. Gollub, M.D., Ph.D.

The tremendous advances in noninvasive brain-imaging technology described in this volume have the potential to aid clinicians in the diagnosis of psychiatric illness and to guide and monitor treatment of psychiatric disease. Several attributes of functional magnetic resonance imaging (fMRI) suggest that this particular imaging modality will be critically important to the realization of this potential. These attributes include safety, reliability, and high spatial and relatively high temporal resolution across the entire brain. One critically important consequence of these attributes is that it is feasible for subjects to be imaged repeatedly over time, thus greatly expanding the range of longitudinal study designs that can directly assess the pathophysiology of psychiatric symptoms. The power of fMRI to reveal information about the function of the brain is greatly increased by integrating fMRI data collected during an experimental paradigm with data collected during an identical paradigm with other imaging tools that have greater temporal resolution, such as electroencephalography (EEG) or magnetoencephalography

(MEG)—a strategy known as multimodal integration. These attributes of fMRI allow the clinician-scientist to probe, in awake, active human subjects, the complex neuronal systems that form the substrate for normal and disordered cognition, emotion, and behavior.

fMRI uses no ionizing radiation, and there are no other known harmful effects of imaging performed within U.S. Food and Drug Administration (FDA)–approved guidelines; thus, fMRI can be repeated safely with individual subjects over time. Importantly, investigators have demonstrated a high degree of consistency in the detected locations of brain activity in individual healthy subjects participating in serial scanning sessions and in healthy subject groups studied across different laboratories when the same experimental paradigm is employed. This consistency suggests that investigators will be able to study within-subject changes in patterns of brain activity related to clinical state (e.g., subjects with bipolar disorder could potentially be imaged while performing the same cognitive task during euthymic, depressed, and manic phases of illness). Similarly, it will be possible to follow changes in brain activity during the progression from symptom exacerbation to remission. And this means that developmental changes in patterns of brain activity can be studied in both healthy and neuropsychiatrically ill subjects. It is important to note, however, that when compared with matched healthy cohorts, psychiatric populations are frequently found to have a marked increase in the variance in fMRI results, including measures of test–retest reliability. This increased variance is likely to be of clinical significance and is deserving of direct investigation.

At the field strength of typical magnetic resonance research magnets (1.5 tesla [T] to 3 T), it is quite a straightforward matter to collect image data from the entire brain. The value of whole-brain mapping is that in addition to testing hypotheses generated from animal research and functional localization studies correlating brain lesions with impairments in function, investigators can detect previously unsuspected brain activity associated with a cognitive, emotional, or behavioral task. Identification of the more widespread network of involved brain regions is especially critical to the study of psychiatric illness that is not necessarily a result of fixed or discrete lesions. For example, multiple groups of investigators in recent fMRI studies of working memory in schizophrenia have identified subtle shifts in specific subregions of the prefrontal cortex, as well as recruitment of subcortical basal ganglia structures, in patients with schizophrenia, compared with matched healthy control subjects.

The spatial resolution of typical fMRI data is on the order of millimeters (mm), even for whole-brain mapping. This resolution increases with higher field strength, at the cost of a more restricted field of view (partial-brain mapping), and is likely to improve over time as imaging technology advances. With currently available spatial resolutions, mapping of activity in the cortex is absolutely feasible, at a level of precision that is close to what a neuropathologist can achieve in postmortem specimens. Such mapping is considerably more difficult in subcortical and brain-stem structures, where functional units (nuclei) are smaller. Despite providing limited information on subcortical structures, the spatial resolutions achievable in current studies are still highly relevant for psychiatrists, given the clear association between cortical dysfunction and many neuropsychiatric symptoms.

Neurons, the basic unit of brain function, have resolvable activity in the millisecond range. By contrast, the temporal resolution of fMRI data is on the order of seconds. The temporal resolution of fMRI is an essential consequence of the fact that measured fMRI signals are the hemodynamic response to changes in neuronal activity. However, with proper attention to experimental design, it is quite feasible to use the temporal resolution of fMRI data to distinguish the functional interplay within brain regions that comprise a network. And by employing the latest technology to obtain—either simultaneously or sequentially—matching electrical recordings (EEG or MEG) and performing multimodal integration analysis, it is possible to elucidate cortical spatiotemporal dynamics of the finest scale. The first such studies in healthy subjects are beginning to emerge; the translation toward clinical utility will follow.

Increasing numbers of studies are using neuroimaging modalities to probe psychiatric illness. To intelligently assess the strengths and weaknesses of these new studies, the practicing psychiatric clinician must have a fundamental understanding of how fMRI studies are designed, implemented, and analyzed. Such knowledge is especially valuable today, a period during which brain-imaging technology is rapidly evolving with respect to methods of data acquisition and analysis. Our goal in this chapter is to acquaint the reader with the basic terminology and concepts involved in the conduct of fMRI studies. We seek to provide a clear explanation and critical appraisal of the fMRI data acquisition, analysis, and experimental design methods most commonly employed in studies of cognition, emotion, and behavior. Most of the published fMRI studies have been performed with cohorts of healthy subjects. A number of fMRI studies have also been conducted in cohorts with psychiatric illness. At present, most of these studies are confined to the realm of investigating the neurobiological mechanism underlying specific symptoms (e.g., auditory hallucinations or working memory deficits in schizophrenia) and have not yet reached a level of maturation required for clinical utility as diagnostic or prognostic markers.

It is worth noting here that functional neuroimaging provides a powerful bridge between the fields of neurology and psychiatry. The greatest gains in knowledge from use of these tools will come from individuals or groups that incorporate all that is known about both the structure and function of the brain in the experimental design and analysis of neuroimaging data.

Basic Physical Principles

The detection of the physical phenomenon known as nuclear magnetic resonance (NMR) can be combined with a technology called magnetic resonance imaging (MRI) to create three-dimensional pictures of the human brain. Conventional MRI creates structural images of the brain at high spatial resolution (typically 1 mm × 1 mm × 1 mm). fMRI, in this context, refers to the detection of changes in blood flow, or blood oxygenation, that are triggered by neural events; these changes are typically imaged at lower spatial resolution. Chapter 2 in this volume describes basic principles of NMR and MRI. Although these are briefly reviewed in the following subsection, the emphasis here is on the specifics of fMRI. (See the Annotated Bibliography at the end of this chapter for pointers to more detailed accounts of the technology.)

Brief Review of NMR and MRI

Prior to generation of the NMR signal, the subject is first placed within a strong magnetic field. This aligns a fraction of the hydrogen nuclei (single protons) in the body. Application of a radio frequency (RF) pulse of magnetic energy, presented at the frequency of the *precession* (i.e., the resonant frequency) of the hydrogen nuclei in water molecules, causes all of those nuclei to change orientation relative to the strong magnetic field. This change in orientation of the nuclei causes the net magnetization to precess around an axis parallel to the main magnet, thus generating a sinusoidally oscillating electric current in a coil of wire placed around the subject's head. This oscillating current is the source of what is called the *NMR signal.*

The NMR signal decays over time for several reasons. First, the protons slowly (on a time scale of seconds for most brain tissue) realign with the main field in the magnet. This realignment is called *longitudinal relaxation,* and the time constant associated with this exponential process is called *T1.* Second, the signal generated by the collection of precessing protons is weakened by the fact that each individual proton experiences a slightly different local magnetic field as a result of interactions with nearby water molecules and other biological tissues, and thus precesses at a frequency slightly different from that of its neighbors. Consequently, these precessing protons fall out of phase with each other (typically on a time scale of tenths of seconds for most brain tissue), so that their respective magnetic fields are no longer lined up and therefore do not generate a detectable, macroscopic signal in the surrounding coil of wire. This aspect of NMR signal decay is sometimes called the "spin-spin component of transverse relaxation," because it is based

on the interaction of the spins (which imply magnetic fields) of nearby nuclei.

If the magnetic field were perfectly uniform, the net decay rate of the signal would be equal to the exponential decay rate, *T2,* which is driven by the combination of spin-spin transverse relaxation and the T1 longitudinal component. (In the brain tissue of interest, T2 is almost entirely determined by the spin-spin relaxation rather than the longitudinal component.) In reality, there are other sources of magnetic field nonuniformity. Imperfections in the main field of the magnet and variations in the magnetic susceptibilities of the different parts of the human body that have been placed within the magnetic field contribute to nonuniformities in the magnetic field experienced by the precessing protons. Most important for fMRI, some chemicals that occur naturally in the body also distort the magnetic field. Deoxyhemoglobin is such a molecule, and because its local concentration varies, the amount of distortion also varies. The rate of exponential decay of the NMR signal is influenced by all of these factors.

Neural Activation, Contrast, and fMRI

Anything causing a change in the NMR signal in a given voxel relative to other voxels at the same time is a source of *image contrast.* In an analogous fashion, changes in the NMR signal at a fixed voxel at different times are interpreted as *functional contrast.* Changing hemodynamics, coupled with the flexibility of MRI, has permitted the detection of functional contrast in three different ways. Historically, changes in *blood volume* were used as a source of contrast in the first human fMRI study. Today, two other hemodynamically based contrast mechanisms are used in studies of neural activation: the first depends on detecting changes in *blood flow,* and the second depends on detecting changes in *blood oxygenation.* These three contrast mechanisms—blood volume, flow, and oxygenation—and their relation to MRI are described in the following paragraphs.

In the earliest fMRI studies, exogenous contrast agents—chemicals injected into the bloodstream of the subject, such as gadolinium—were used to enhance contrast. These bloodborne chemicals produced local distortions in the magnetic field, thus allowing increases in cerebral blood volume to be detected. Subsequent studies demonstrated that endogenous contrast agents (i.e., naturally occurring molecules in the body, such as deoxyhemoglobin in the blood) could also yield sufficient contrast between different states of neural activity. The use of endogenous contrast agents obviated the need for injecting foreign molecules into the bodies of healthy subjects, and this is one of the key reasons that fMRI has become so popular as a technique for assessing human brain function.

When neurons are active in a region of brain, blood flow and blood volume local to that region of activity increase. The idea is that when fresh blood flows into the slice of the brain that is being imaged, it will have a different "spin history" (i.e., it will not have recently been struck by an orientation-flipping RF pulse) and thus will have a greater degree of alignment with the main field in the magnet. When another RF pulse is applied, the fresh blood will have a greater concentration of aligned protons to flip and therefore will yield a greater NMR signal. Because the imaging of this signal occurs on a time scale that is rapid with respect to the blood flow, the change is detected. This phenomenon is the basis for "flow-based" imaging in fMRI. It is largely sensitive to changes in arterial blood flow (where flow is the fastest).

A second—and more commonly used—process also yields a fMRI signal. Surprisingly, the neural activity that elicited the local increase in blood flow and blood volume does not elicit a proportional increase in oxygen utilization. That is, although the neural activity leads to a small increase in oxygen utilization, that increase is dwarfed by the increase in blood flow. Thus, an increase in oxygenated hemoglobin occurs in the venous portion of the capillary bed near the site of neural activity (as well as downstream from that site). The combination of increased oxygenated hemoglobin and increased blood flow results in a *decrease* in the instantaneous concentration of deoxygenated hemoglobin on the venous side of the capillaries. Deoxygenated hemoglobin (unlike oxygenated hemoglobin) is a strongly paramagnetic biological molecule, and it distorts the magnetic field locally. Thus, a *decrease* in the local concentration of deoxyhemoglobin leads to a more uniform magnetic field locally and to a longer time period during which the orientations of precessing protons remain in phase. As a result, the NMR signal from a brain region of reduced deoxyhemoglobin concentration *increases* relative to the signal from that brain region in its normal (neuronally resting) state. This link between changes in neuronal activity and changes in the localized blood oxygenation is what gives rise to the fMRI signal change, a phenomenon called the blood oxygen level–dependent (BOLD) effect. This effect is the major source of contrast in most fMRI experiments. The mechanism underlying the coupling of neuronal activity (e.g., neuronal "spiking," synaptic potentials, main-

tenance of resting potentials) to the hemodynamic response is the subject of active investigation (for further information, see the Annotated Bibliography at the end of this chapter).

Other Technical Issues in MRI

Operationally, fMRI differs from conventional MRI in two basic respects. First, fMRI is tailored to be sensitive to changes in blood flow and/or oxygenation that reflect neural activity. Second, fMRI is typically conducted with special hardware that permits the very rapid variation of magnetic field gradients that is needed to create images. This rapid variation of gradients permits much faster acquisition of whole-brain volumes than is possible with conventional MRI. This swift data collection is crucial in most modern fMRI-based experiments, as will become apparent in the discussion of experimental design and data analysis.

Several imaging parameters must be selected during acquisition and should be optimized for each study. Figure 4–1 illustrates some of the advantages of optimizing acquisition parameters for fMRI scans. The figure compares the results from an experimental paradigm conducted twice with the same individual using two different sets of acquisition parameters. The studies sought to characterize the pattern of brain activity associated with the euphoriogenic effects of the abused substance cocaine (the references for these studies are provided in the Annotated Bibliography). One subject participated in two separate experiments. The first study was conducted at a field strength of 1.5 T with 6-mm-thick slices collected every 8 seconds. A second study to replicate and extend the first was conducted at a higher field strength (3 T) with thinner image slices (3 mm thick) collected more frequently over time (repetition time [TR]=4 seconds). The combination of higher field strength, thinner slices, and more timepoints provided sufficient power to allow the investigators to analyze the data for individual subjects rather than being limited to group analyses.

fMRI is made practical and powerful by virtue of special pulse sequences (e.g., echo planar and spiral scanning) and hardware that permit the encoding of a brain slice with a single RF pulse, allowing the entire brain to be imaged in a matter of a few seconds. A wide variety of pulse sequences are used in fMRI, and pulse-sequence development remains an area of continuing innovation. Moreover, the versatility of MRI for neuroscience extends beyond fMRI; magnetic resonance can also be used to assay various aspects of brain chemistry

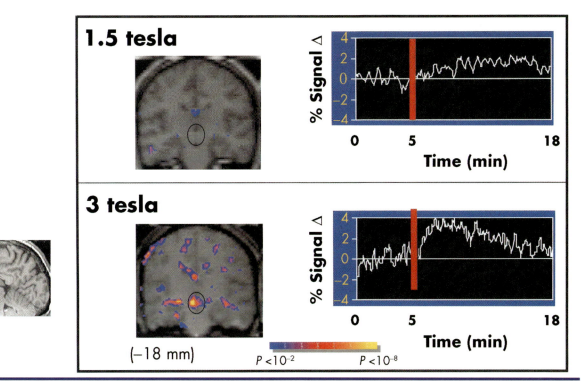

Figure 4–1. Effect of image acquisition parameters on functional magnetic resonance imaging (fMRI) signal. *Top* and *bottom* panel each show representative data from a single substance-abusing subject who participated in two similar studies of the effects of acute cocaine infusion on brain activity (see Annotated Bibliography for a complete account of the studies and results). One study was conducted with a 1.5-tesla (T) magnet, and the other with a 3-T magnet. For each study, a pseudocolored statistical map showing significant fMRI signal changes after cocaine infusion is superimposed on a gray-scale anatomic image of a coronal slice through the brain at a level 18 mm posterior to the anterior commissure. Kolmogorov-Smirnov statistical maps compare the pre- and postinfusion time points. Adjacent to that image is shown the time course of fMRI signal change (the infusion is indicated by the *red line*) in the cluster of voxels located in the ventral tegmental region of the brain (delimited by the *black oval*). Note that the fMRI acquisition parameters for the 1.5-T study had few time points and thicker slices. The improved power from the 3-T study allowed the investigators to probe brain activity of individual subjects, not just group-averaged data. The *black line* on the small sagittal image indicates the approximate slice plane.
Source. Data from Breiter et al. 1997; Gollub et al. 1998, 1999 (see Annotated Bibliography).

by means of a technique known as magnetic resonance spectroscopy (MRS). Because some variants of MRS can measure the presence of brain metabolites at temporal resolutions on the order of minutes and spatial resolutions not far from those of BOLD fMRI, MRS is in many ways conceptually related to fMRI and is likely to have increasing clinical applications in psychiatry in the future (see Chapter 5 in this volume).

Summary of Basic Physical Principles

A strong, spatially uniform magnetic field aligns a small but significant fraction of the hydrogen nuclei of water molecules in a brain. A carefully controlled sequence of gradient fields and RF pulses is used to generate NMR signals that can be reconstructed to form a three-dimensional image in which contrast is dependent, in part, on the blood flow and/or oxygenation changes caused by neural activity. Thus, fMRI can be used noninvasively to detect changes in local neural activity in the human brain.

Research Methods

Consideration of experimental design in the context of fMRI-based studies is inextricably associated with data analysis. We begin the following discussion by reviewing some basic issues in experimental design, and then describe related issues in data analysis. Fundamental to the understanding of fMRI as a tool for representing the localization of brain function is the idea that a single image, in isolation, conveys little, if any, useful information. Rather, it is the comparison of multiple images that are collected during different states of neural activity that supplies interpretable data. Note that this statement is not true for structural MR images. A single structural image conveys a great deal of useful information, because data about change are not sought (except on a much longer time scale, as in developmental and longitudinal studies of brain structure). In contrast, functional imaging data is almost exclusively about changes in neuronal activity. Moreover, although changes between two brain states can be detected with fMRI, the interpretation of those changes normally requires additional measurements of brain states or other prior knowledge. For example, merely observing that the fMRI signal is larger for a specific brain region during task 1 than it is during task 2 does not allow one to determine whether the signal increase represents an "activation" of neural activity by task 1 or an "inhibition" of neural activity by task 2. Comparison with other states (e.g., a resting baseline of some sort) is needed to disambiguate the interpretation of the data.

Experimental Design

The design of fMRI-based experimental paradigms is influenced by a number of considerations. The spatial and temporal characteristics of the blood flow response underlying the fMRI BOLD signal place limitations on the kinds of neural effects that can be studied and also strongly influence the way in which specific experiments or test procedures must be arranged. Practical constraints associated with fMRI derive from the requirements (typically) for long imaging sessions, minimal head movement throughout the session, tolerance of the much louder acoustic noise associated with high-speed imaging, and the need to present stimuli and obtain behavioral responses. Finally, it is essential to understand that fMRI is a tool that depends on the comparison of multiple brain states rather than a snapshot of a single state.

fMRI is dependent on hemodynamic changes rather than the electrical consequences of neural activity. The spatial and temporal characteristics of these hemodynamic effects must be taken into account in designing experiments and analyzing the data from these experiments. The spatial characteristics arise from the underlying vasculature and details (as yet unknown) of biochemical coupling between neuronal activity and hemodynamic response; the temporal characteristics

include a delay in the onset of detectable MR signal changes in response to neural activity and a dispersion of the resulting hemodynamic changes over a longer time than the initiating neural events.

Block Design

With regard to the temporal aspects of the hemodynamics measured, fMRI experiments fall into two broad categories: "block" designs and "event-related" designs. In block designs, the experimental task is performed continuously in blocks of time, typically 20–60 seconds in duration. The idea here is to ignore the details of the temporal characteristics by setting up a "steady state" of neuronal and hemodynamic change. This approach is conceptually simple and is of great practical importance for fMRI, because it is the optimal technique for detecting small changes in brain activity. The major weakness of block design is the requirement that all the stimuli or task characteristics remain unchanged for tens of seconds, precluding the use of many classic psychological paradigms (e.g., the "oddball" scheme).

Event-Related Design

The other major approach—event-related design—makes use of the details of the temporal response pattern in the hemodynamics, as well as the largely linear response characteristics associated with multiple stimulus presentations. Many instances of each of a small number of stimulus types are presented in a pseudorandom order (rather than in blocks of similar or identical stimulus types), and the hemodynamic response to each stimulus type is extracted. The associated data analysis is more difficult than in the case of block design, because the hemodynamic responses to the different stimulus presentations overlap in time. Nonetheless, single-trial designs are particularly powerful and useful in circumstances in which it is essential to have random order in the presentation of individual stimuli—that is, in a situation in which a block design with long periods of the same type of stimulus would not permit the desired comparisons for neural activations.

Time-Resolved Design

One final approach to experimental design should be mentioned. The techniques described thus far make use of averaging over multiple instances of a given stimulus type. In block designs, the trials of a given type all occur together, so the averaging is done as much by the hemodynamics and neural systems as by any data analysis software. In event-related designs, the averaging of the effects of multiple stimulus presentations of a given type is done explicitly in software during data analysis. It is possible, however, to analyze spaced single-trial data on the basis of activation from a single event (rather than averaging over multiple instances of the same trial type). This technique—sometimes called time-resolved fMRI—has not yet been widely applied, primarily because the signals elicited from single stimulus events are generally weak. However, high–magnetic field MRI systems and selection of experimental paradigms that elicit strong, focal neural activity have demonstrated the feasibility of single-event fMRI.

Tradeoffs

The key physical variables associated with fMRI—spatial resolution, temporal resolution, brain coverage, and signal-to-noise ratio—are quantities whose values can be manipulated by trading one off against the others. The physiology of the circulatory system and the physics of the MR imaging devices constrain the spatial and temporal resolution of fMRI. It is routine, today, to obtain 1 mm × 1 mm × 1 mm structural MR images and 5 mm × 5 mm × 5 mm functional MR images in 1.5-T devices. The temporal resolution of fMRI is on the order of 1–3 seconds. Neither the spatial- nor the temporal-resolution numbers are indicative of absolute limits in terms of the physiology or the imaging hardware. Rather, these numbers represent a snapshot in the development of ever-improving resolutions. Moreover, at any given stage of technical development in MRI, the various imaging parameters can be manipulated to emphasize one aspect of resolution in exchange for another.

Practical Constraints

The physical properties of MRI, as well as financial costs, place a number of practical constraints on the design and execution of fMRI-based studies, thereby influencing experimental design. Subjects must be screened for disqualifying conditions (e.g., presence of a cardiac pacemaker, claustrophobia), ancillary equipment must be MR-compatible, and financial resources to support the imaging acquisition must be available.

Head Movement

One vexing problem in the practical application of fMRI is head movement. Although pulse sequences have been developed that allow collection of an entire slice of brain data in less than 50 milliseconds, and multiple slices (for whole-brain coverage) can be collected in 2–3 seconds, the amount of information contained in each such image is limited. That is, the amount of functional contrast in the images—the differences in the signals between two experimental states—is small. To make up for this limitation, many images are collected over extended periods of time: at least minutes, and sometimes hours. During these time periods, it is important that the subject's head move as little as possible.

Subject movement is generally regarded as the greatest obstacle to obtaining consistent data in fMRI-based experiments. A variety of techniques are used to encourage subjects to keep their heads as still as possible, but none of these is perfect. With young, well-motivated, healthy subjects, head movement is usually not an insurmountable problem. Studies with experienced, well-motivated subjects who use bite bars (an individually molded dental impression mounted to the head coil) in the scanner can routinely be expected to yield data free of serious motion artifact. By contrast, in studies with psychiatric patients (e.g., schizophrenia patients or substance-abusing subjects who cannot use a bite bar because they have few, if any, teeth), older patients, or other difficult subjects, as much as 20%–30% of the data may need to be discarded because of subject motion. Although data analytic procedures are available for transforming images of moving heads back to a fixed position, these procedures are limited. Indeed, because the moving head actually distorts the main magnetic field in different ways, no motion-correction algorithm can fix the problem completely.

Finally, it should be noted that MRI time is expensive. Charges for an hour of clinical imaging can run to the hundreds of dollars. Therefore, the total number of imaging minutes is one of the parameters that must be considered in the tradeoffs when designing a study. At the same time, the research field is recognizing that results based on small sample sizes can be erroneous or misleading; therefore, having adequate resources to study a full cohort of at least 15–18 subjects is critical to obtaining interpretable (and publishable) data.

Data Analysis

The scanning session for a typical fMRI-based experiment lasts 1–3 hours and results in the collection of hundreds of megabytes of data. The theory and practicalities associated with processing those data are complex and continually evolving. The present spatial and temporal resolution of fMRI data encourages modeling of brain systems at a level that may substantially exceed that of previous volumetric imaging systems. Some of these advances require different kinds of data analysis and different kinds of visualization tools than made sense in the context of systems with poorer spatial resolution. Finally, the ability to image the same subject multiple times, and the associated potential for collection of many kinds of functional data from that subject, encourages novel approaches to data analysis.

Data analysis is a critical, still time-consuming, and at times controversial part of fMRI-based experimentation. Although many of the problems are well defined, the appropriate solutions are not. There is general agreement on how to handle some of the issues associated with data analysis (e.g., algorithms to detect and correct for head movement), but there are no universally agreed upon approaches to many other issues (e.g., the appropriate statistical tests to define the detection of neural activation, the best way to compare data across different subjects, the best way to visualize and report the results of data analysis). A host of software tools are available for data analysis, each having particular strengths and weaknesses. Because of the rapid development in all aspects of fMRI-based research, no one standard approach to data analysis has yet emerged.

Preprocessing

Before the essential part of data analysis can begin, a number of preliminary steps are typically taken. The most critical of these is assessment of head movement. In many new MRI systems, some measure of head movement is computed during the scanning session after each run; in at least one system, the imaging software itself performs prospective slice correction, resetting the imaging parameters in real time (during the scanning run) to compensate for detected movement between the previous volumetric images.

The data analytic approach to motion detection and motion correction is based on the brain images themselves, rather than on the external monitoring of head movement. Efforts are made to minimize subject head movement, but it is not currently possible to correct for severe or rapid movement. (All of the current algorithms for correcting head movement assume rigid motion of the head. Whereas a single slice of brain-imaging data is collected very rapidly relative to most head movement, the time needed to collect an entire brain volume—consisting of 20 or more slices—is much longer than many head movements. Such motion cannot be corrected with these algorithms.) However, if

the movement is not too great in amplitude and not too rapid, the algorithms available in most fMRI data analysis packages are adequate to detect the motion and to transform the data to compensate for the effects of that motion.

A key feature of these algorithms is that they automatically reveal many kinds of movement, including stimulus-correlated movement. If the subject moves every time he or she is supposed to start a task, the movement could create MRI signal artifacts that appear as a false activation signal. There is no good way to correct for such data; it must be detected and discarded.

Basic Detection of Change

The first goals of any analysis of fMRI-based data are to determine whether the experimental manipulation has resulted in a measurable change in the MR signal and, if so, to specify where (in the brain) and when (in time) that change has occurred. In principle, any statistical method that can be applied to a time series can be used with fMRI data. In practice, the demands of the experimental paradigm, the limitations of the tool, and the capabilities of the distributed software packages constrain the sorts of analyses that are typically performed. A few broad classes of common data analysis options are detailed in the following discussion (this list is not comprehensive). With the exception of principal components analysis (PCA) and other multivariate techniques, each of these tests is applied at the voxel level. When these statistics are computed for each voxel in the brain and the resulting collection of statistics is presented in the form of an image in which color or intensity is used to represent the value of that statistic, the result is called a "statistical map" of brain activation.

Systematic Detection of Change

The most obvious and simple statistical test that can be used in fMRI data analysis is Student's t test. This test assumes that each number in each group is independent and that the underlying distribution of numbers is Gaussian (i.e., it is a parametric test). In fact, both of these assumptions are often violated in actual fMRI data. Nonetheless, parametric statistics such as the t test are the most widely used measures of the difference between the groups of numbers collected in fMRI images across conditions.

The mathematical machinery used to compute t tests and other variants on correlation analysis with fMRI data is the general linear model. The fMRI data are compared with some kind of reference temporal function to determine in which brain regions the fMRI signal intensity is highly correlated with a collection of reference functions. Most candidate reference functions are obtained from the experimental design. For example, because the brain's hemodynamic response assumes a fairly consistent profile (delayed in onset and longer lasting relative to the inciting stimulus), a boxcar function defining the experimental paradigm is often convolved with an estimated hemodynamic response function to yield the reference function. The resulting reference function is smoother than a boxcar and better takes into account the shape of the hemo-dynamic response, generally resulting in better corre-lation between the MR signal time courses and the regressor time course. Often, a single canonical hemo-dynamic response function is used across the entire brain and across subjects, despite the fact that evi-dence exists for variation in hemodynamic response shape across subjects and brain regions. Some soft-ware packages make provisions for this variation, allowing for independent modeling of the hemo-dynamic response function on a voxelwise basis. Fig-ure 4–2 shows brain activation related to a working-memory task as "seen by" the hemodynamic response in the dorsolateral prefrontal cortex of a subject with schizophrenia.

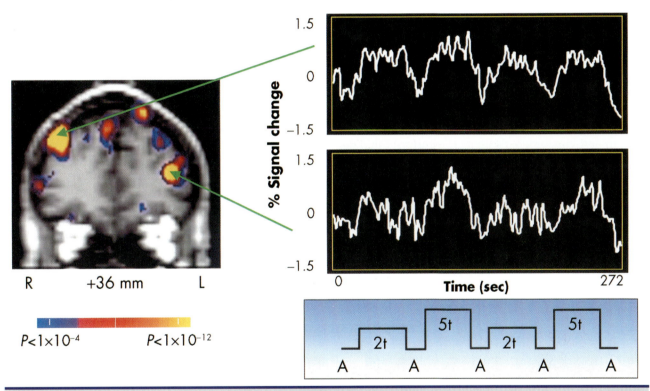

Figure 4–2.　Statistical map showing bilateral dorsolateral prefrontal cortex activation in an unmedicated sub-ject with schizophrenia during performance of the Sternberg Item Recognition Paradigm, a task that requires working memory to function to obtain better-than-chance performance.

The *t*-test statistical map was generated by comparing the images acquired during the five-target (5t) condition with those acquired during the Arrows (A) baseline condition. The task paradigm is depicted graphically below the time course of signal intensity changes (see Annotated Bibliography for a complete account of the study and results). Note the marked differences between the right and left side in the activation produced by the easier condition (two targets [2t]).

Source.　Data from Manoach et al. 2000 (see Annotated Bibliography).

All of the approaches discussed thus far make the assumption that the variations of interest in the data are those that occur in temporal synchrony with the ex-perimental variations built into the design and that these variations can be modeled at individual voxels in the image data (i.e., they are *univariate* techniques). This is by far the most commonly used method of data analysis. Other approaches (e.g., principal components analysis, independent components analysis, partial least squares, structural equation modeling) go beyond this simple approach to try to find and understand spatiotemporal patterns of activation that are not based on the isolated time course at a single voxel. Such tests should be able to detect novel temporal variations triggered by the experiment but not part of the design. However, routine analysis of fMRI-based data in clinical contexts will probably not be based on these multivariate techniques in the near future.

Comparing Brains

Clinical applications require the ability to make sense of data from an *individual* brain. In contrast, most experimental and validation studies must have some system for comparing brains across subjects. Nearly all fMRI studies use multiple subjects and perform statistical analyses across data collected from multiple subjects. Brains differ in size, shape, and details of sulcal/gyral folding. Various systems have been developed to "spatially normalize" the brains—that is, to transform the images to a coordinate system that will permit comparison across subjects. Systems for performing such transformations range from the very basic (e.g., each brain is set in a standard orientation and linearly scaled to fit in a standard rectangular box) to the highly elaborate (e.g., the cortical surface is treated as a rubber sheet that can be inflated to smooth out sulci and gyri, thus permitting easy visualization of cortex within the folds, as well as on the surface).

Comparing Groups

In addition to comparing brains across individual subjects in a given group, researchers often try to detect and understand differences between groups. fMRI can be used to address at least two types of questions. One question might be thought of as the attempt to represent "typical" brain function and associated networks of activity. In that context, collecting more and more data about a single brain engaged in a single task might be useful, because the variability associated with any particular aspect of the associated brain activity might be expected to decrease with increased measurement. In statistics, this is called a "fixed effects" model. On the other hand, to know whether there are differences in brain function and networks of activity between two putatively different groups of subjects, it is important to sample many members of each group, even if the individual measurement of any one mem-

ber of the group has low precision. In particular, knowing with extreme precision that two members of one group differ from two members of another group is useful only if the within-group variation (i.e., between brains) is as small as the within-brain variation (i.e., between multiple measurements of the same brain). If this is not the case, the exceptional precision of the measurement of the small number of subjects is not useful. In statistics, this is known as a "random effects" model.

The practical implication of the fixed- versus random-effects model of variance for functional neuroimaging is that it is better to have measurements of many brains if the goal is to claim group differences. On the other hand, it may be better to have many measurements of a few brains if the goal is to delineate functional systems as precisely as possible.

Software Tools

Many software tools are available for analyzing data from fMRI. Some are completely free (e.g., AFNI, FSL, FreeSurfer), others are mostly free (SPM is "free" but requires a MATLAB license, which is not free), and still others are supported by commercial ventures (e.g., Analyze, MEDx, BrainVoyager). MRI manufacturers are beginning to incorporate fMRI analysis software with their scanners, a practice that will undoubtedly increase in the near future. Development of these data analysis systems is rapid and ongoing; up-to-date information is best and most easily obtained via the World Wide Web. One particularly exciting development is that of real-time fMRI data analysis capability. It is now possible to perform a simple statistical test on fMRI data during the experiment (while the participant is still in the MRI scanner) that tells the investigator whether a successful fMRI study has been obtained. Such a test can be of significant practical value, for two reasons. First, if analysis reveals excessive head movement or other artifact, an additional run can be obtained on the spot, without having to bring the subject back to the MRI suite at a later date. Second, it is possible to increase efficiency by repeating a given activation protocol only as long as is necessary to detect any effects at a given (operator-specified) threshold for statistical significance.

Summary of Research Methods

The decisions required in the design of a useful fMRI experiment and the choice of appropriate data analysis methods are intertwined and complex. Application of the technology of fMRI to psychiatry entails a collection of tradeoffs. The 10 years since the inception of fMRI have seen dramatic developments in the technology underlying image acquisition as well as in methods for experimental design and data analysis. Today, an array of established procedures and software tools are available with which to implement these ideas, although no universally accepted standards yet exist. A simple, systematic set of neuropsychological test procedures appropriate for the study of psychiatric illnesses, including standardized data analyses, is undoubtedly on its way, but it has not yet arrived.

Potential Clinical Applications

fMRI has many possible clinical applications. A very active current area of research is the use of fMRI for presurgical planning for patients with brain tumors or epilepsy. fMRI's greatest potential may lie in the areas of differential diagnosis and treatment evaluation. One illustration of this potential can be found in a recent study of the detailed process of "spreading depression" in neural activity associated with migraine headaches and their associated visual sequelae (Hadjikhani et al. 2001). In that study, fMRI permitted the investigators to follow the progression of the vasoconstrictive events systematically across the visual cortex. The potential for such applications in the context of differential diagnosis and treatment evaluation is obvious.

A tour de force in fMRI-based experimentation, the study of Hadjikhani and colleagues (2001) brought together some of the most elegant work ever conducted in a research application context (retinotopic mapping of the visual cortex) with a phenomenon of long-standing clinical importance (migraine headaches). Migraines are an intense form of headache that often is preceded by visual auras—that is, the perception of various strange visual patterns, typically around a circular arc or perimeter of some portion of the visual field, bilaterally—and an associated temporary blindness (a temporary scotoma) within that perimeter. The fact that these auras and scotomas appear to both eyes at the same portion of the visual field is very strong suggestive evidence that the underlying effect is being controlled at the cortical level—where these corresponding portions of the visual field share the same physical location in the brain. Moreover, migraines have long been understood to be associated with

changes in dilation and constriction of the cerebral vasculature.

Migraine headache is very difficult to study with fMRI, both because the aura phenomenon is relatively short-lived (sometimes 30–60 minutes, sometimes 2–4 hours) and because the headache is associated with aversion to loud noises and bright lights on the part of the sufferer. Therefore, it is difficult to persuade migraine patients to volunteer for an fMRI study; and even if they were willing, it would be rare for such subjects to experience a migraine while they were near the scanner. One research group was fortunate enough to find a volunteer who predictably and regularly triggered his own migraine headache by engaging in intense athletic activity (playing basketball). He was, therefore, available for repeated (schedulable!) scanning immediately before and during the onset of his migraine attacks.

The investigators, experts in visual retinotopy, designed a protocol that revealed—in exquisite detail—the neurological correlates of the patient's visual symptoms. As the scotoma grew and as the aura changed in size (both of which phenomena could be reported subjectively by the patient), fMRI data revealed the location on the cortex and the functional variation in amplitude of response to a flickering checkerboard of visual stimulation. Combining these data with previously obtained retinotopic maps of the subject's visual cortex permitted a precise correlation between measurable function and subjective vision loss. Although this study does not directly suggest a treatment for migraine attacks, it certainly demonstrates a method for objectively assessing the effectiveness of candidate therapies.

Conclusions

Many factors suggest that fMRI will make critically important contributions to the diagnostic and prognostic capabilities of future psychiatrists. The first of these is the rapid evolution of the technology for fMRI image acquisition, which allows ever-greater spatial and temporal resolution. The second factor is advances in experimental design and data analysis tools. Finally, increasingly sophisticated approaches to data modeling that utilize calibrated imaging data in conjunction with other clinical information, including genomics, in large-scale multisite projects will begin to reveal the dysfunction in neural activity that underlies psychiatric illness.

Annotated Bibliography

For a much more thorough and elegant explanation of the physics underlying magnetic resonance (MR) image formation, blood oxygen level–dependent (BOLD) contrast, and other MR signals, the interested reader is referred to the following textbook:

Buxton RB: Introduction to Functional Magnetic Resonance Imaging: Principles and Techniques. Cambridge, UK, Cambridge University Press, 2002

For more details on the practicalities of setting up experiments in the magnetic resonance imaging (MRI) environment, experimental paradigm design, and data analysis, the reader is referred to the appropriate chapters in the following textbook:

Jezzard P, Matthews PM, Smith SM (eds): Functional MRI: An Introduction to Methods. Oxford, UK, Oxford University Press, 2001

And to the following:

Friston KJ, Holmes AP, Worsley KJ: How many subjects constitute a study? Neuroimage 10:1–5, 1999

Gusnard DA, Raichle ME: Searching for a baseline: functional imaging and the resting human brain. Nat Rev Neurosci 2:685–694, 2001

Manoach DS: Prefrontal cortex dysfunction during working memory performance in schizophrenia: reconciling discrepant findings. Schizophr Res 60:285–298, 2003

Stark CE, Squire LR: When zero is not zero: the problem of ambiguous baseline conditions in fMRI. Proc Natl Acad Sci U S A 98:12760–12766, 2001

For more information regarding the coupling of neuronal activity with changes in cerebral vasculature, the reader is referred to the relevant chapters in the textbooks listed above and, for even greater detail, the appropriate chapters in the following textbook:

Edvinsson L, Krause D (eds): Cerebral Blood Flow and Metabolism, 2nd Edition. Philadelphia, PA, Lippincott, Williams & Wilkins, 2002

For a practical demonstration of issues regarding test–retest reliability in psychiatric populations, see the following:

Manoach DS, Halpern EF, Kramer TS, et al: Test-retest reliability of a functional MRI working memory paradigm in normal and schizophrenic subjects. Am J Psychiatry 158:955–958, 2001

For interesting and thoughtful discussions of what has been learned that is relevant to cognitive and emotional aspects of brain function from neuroimaging, see the following:

Bush G, Luu P, Posner MI: Cognitive and emotional influences in anterior cingulate cortex. Trends Cogn Sci 4:215–222, 2000

For a complete description of the migraine study described in the text, see the following:

Hadjikhani N, Sanchez Del Rio M, Wu O, et al: Mechanisms of migraine aura revealed by functional MRI in human visual cortex. Proc Natl Acad Sci U S A 98:4687–4692, 2001

For a full account of the studies on the effects of acute cocaine infusion on human brain activity described in Figure 4–1, see the following:

Breiter H, Gollub RL, Weisskoff RM, et al: Acute effects of cocaine on human brain activity. Neuron 19:591–611, 1997

Gollub RL, Breiter H, Kantor H, et al: Cocaine decreases cortical cerebral blood flow, but does not obscure regional activation in functional magnetic resonance imaging in human subjects. J Cereb Blood Flow Metab 18:724–734, 1998

Gollub RL, Breiter H, Dershwitz M, et al: Cocaine dose dependent activation of brain reward circuitry in humans revealed by 3T fMRI. Paper presented at: 7th Scientific Meeting and Exhibition of the International Society for Magnetic Resonance in Medicine, Philadelphia, PA, May 24–28, 1999

For a complete account of the study from which the data in Figure 4–2 were taken, see the following:

Manoach DS, Gollub RL, Benson EB, et al: Schizophrenia subjects show aberrant fMRI activation of dorsolateral prefrontal cortex and basal ganglia during working memory performance. Biol Psychiatry 48:99–109, 2000

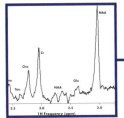

Magnetic Resonance Spectroscopy

Nicolas Bolo, Ph.D.
Perry F. Renshaw, M.D., Ph.D.

Since the discovery of the principle of nuclear magnetic resonance (NMR), the property of atomic nuclei to absorb and emit energy through rapidly oscillating magnetic fields has been used as an investigational tool in domains as widespread as organic or solid state chemistry, geology, molecular biology, and medicine. It is now so familiar to and universal in the medical field that the term magnetic resonance (MR) brings to mind for many an array of methods, techniques, and instrumentation with powerful diagnostic capabilities. Numerous medical specialties have benefited from use of this tool to increase diagnostic power, mostly due to MR's ability to noninvasively capture images that contain structural or functional information from soft tissues deep within the body. The organ of interest for the psychiatrist is the brain. The technique is widely known as magnetic resonance imaging (MRI) for structural MR imaging. But the versatility of MR allows its methods to extend beyond static structure to investigate dynamic processes within a broad range of levels of biological organization, from biochemical pathways of

neurotransmitter synthesis to the integration of cortical functional activity for behavioral responses to stimuli (functional MRI [fMRI] is addressed in Chapter 4). It is generally less well known that brain biochemistry may be explored by an MR method called magnetic resonance spectroscopy (MRS). In this chapter we discuss the clinical utility of MRS methods in psychiatry.

Magnetic Resonance Investigational Methods

Nuclear Magnetic Resonance in Historical Perspective

NMR is a phenomenon that can be found in both living and inorganic matter of our world. One physics textbook offers the following summary: "Magnetic resonance is a phenomenon found in magnetic systems that possess both magnetic moment and angular momentum. A system such as the nucleus of an atom may consist of many particles coupled together so that in any given state, the nucleus possesses a total magnetic moment μ and a total angular momentum J" (Slichter 1996, pp. 1–2). The first NMR experiment—in which NMR signals were detected from a molecular beam of lithium chloride—was performed in 1938. MR experiments in bulk matter followed several years later, in 1946. In 1951, the property that similar nuclei in different molecular structures have slightly different resonant frequencies was demonstrated in experiments performed on samples of ethanol. This property allows for magnetic resonance spectroscopy, or the presentation of the MR signal intensity distribution on a frequency axis, which is widely used in organic chemistry for the determination of molecular structure. The experiments in living systems followed soon after, with some of the first reports on the application of MRS to cells and tissues made in 1955. In 1973, phosphorus-31 (^{31}P) NMR recordings from erythrocytes were reported. By the early 1980s, improvements in MR system design had made it possible to conduct studies in vivo. By 1986, the scientific literature contained reports of ^{31}P MR in vivo studies of brain, kidney, liver, heart, skeletal muscle, and bowel.

Principles of Magnetic Resonance Spectroscopy

Compounds are formed of atoms. Nuclei of atoms with an odd number of *nucleons* (building blocks of the nucleus, composed of positively charged protons and neutral neutrons) are positively charged particles with spin that possess a property called *magnetic moment.* In the classical description, the interaction of the magnetic moment with the static magnetic field of the scanner orients a fraction of the nuclear magnetic moments parallel to the magnetic field, resulting in a sum effect, or *induced magnetization.* The direction of the scanner's magnetic field is called the longitudinal direction, and the plane perpendicular to this field is called the transverse plane. The induced magnetization—which carries information about the compound—is detected by the MR scanner in the transverse plane. A magnetic field that is oscillating at the appropriate resonant frequency of the nucleus drives the induced magnetization into the transverse plane for detection. In the quantum mechanical description at the microscopic level, the magnetization flip corresponds to transitions between energy or coherence states of the nuclei. The main nuclei of interest for biological studies with MR

Table 5–1. Nuclei of biological interest with relative nuclear magnetic resonance (NMR) sensitivities

Nucleus	Spin quantum number	NMR frequency at 4 tesla	Relative sensitivity at constant field	% natural abundance
^{1}H	1/2	170.32	1	99.8
^{19}F	1/2	162.13	0.83	100
^{7}Li	3/2	66.21	0.29	92.58
^{23}Na	3/2	45.04	0.09	100
^{31}P	1/2	69.01	0.06	100
^{13}C	1/2	42.85	0.02	1.1
^{39}K	3/2	7.97	0.0005	93.2

are outlined in Table 5–1, which shows that the resonant frequencies are in the radio frequency (RF) domain.

The resonant frequency depends on two values: the value of an intrinsic property of the nucleus, called the *gyromagnetic ratio,* and the value of the field in which the nucleus bathes, which in principle is the scanner's static magnetic field:

$$\begin{pmatrix} \text{resonant} \\ \text{frequency} \end{pmatrix} = \begin{pmatrix} \text{gyromagnetic} \\ \text{ratio} \end{pmatrix} \times \begin{pmatrix} \text{magnetic} \\ \text{field} \end{pmatrix}$$

The signal is detected at a bandwidth centered on the driving RF field frequency. In a given compound, the distribution of electron clouds around the nuclear backbone creates a shielding effect so that each nucleus may experience a field that is in fact slightly different from the scanner field; thus, the resonant frequency may be slightly different than the driving frequency, depending on the position of the nucleus in the compound's electron cloud. These frequency shifts, called *chemical shifts* because of their chemical origin, are on the order of several to several hundred hertz (Hz), whereas the driving resonant frequency is on the order of several to several hundred million hertz (megahertz [MHz]); thus, frequency shifts are often measured in parts per million (ppm) of the resonant frequency. The frequency analysis of the detected signal or spectrum allows identification of the compound. Each compound has its own "frequency signature" in the MR spectrum. Similar chemical groups or similar electron clouds give rise to resonant frequencies that are close; thus, peak overlap is often encountered in the spectrum. Overcoming this overlap so as to distinguish different chemical entities is one of the difficulties inherent in MRS.

Magnetic Resonance Spectroscopy Relative to Other Neuroimaging Modalities

The other main neuroimaging modalities comparable to MRS, inasmuch as they can also reveal biochemical information from tissues in vivo, are positron emission tomography (PET) and single photon emission computed tomography (SPECT). All of these techniques are noninvasive in the sense that they do not require surgery, but PET and SPECT require the injection of a radioactive marker that is traced by the detector system. Unlike PET and SPECT, MRS can detect endogenous metabolites. Exogenously administered compounds can also be observed with MRS, but they need not be radioactive to be detected by MRS methods. Thus, in contrast to PET and SPECT, MRS allows repeated imaging without the risk of exposure to radioactivity or ionizing radiation: studies of pharmacological kinetics can be performed, as well as longitudinal studies over weeks, months, or years, without the hazard of accumulated radiation effects. Another advantage of MR is that it constitutes a multimodal technique: investigation of several aspects of brain structure, function, and biochemistry can be carried out in a single examination session while the patient is in the scanner. The combined measurement of several MR parameters can be more powerful and informative than single measurements alone.

The main disadvantage of MR is that it has a low sensitivity, requiring relatively high concentrations of the target compound to be present in order to be detected. The consequence of this low sensitivity is the low spatial and temporal resolution of MRS recordings. The signal-to-noise ratio of the MRS recording increases with static magnetic field strength—hence the drive among clinicians and research scientists alike for MR systems with higher and higher fields. At present, the U.S. Food and Drug Administration (FDA) has approved scanners with a field strength of up to 3 tesla (T) for clinical use. In research applications, scanners with fields up to 4 T are in operation; two research sites in the United States currently have FDA approval for human studies at 7 T, and manufacturers are considering yet higher fields. The higher field strength of research scanners provides another advantage over lower–field strength clinical scanners: the spectral spread increases with field strength, thus reducing the overlap between resonance peaks. The increased spectral resolution allows better separation, identification, and quantita-

tion of several metabolites that could not easily be studied at lower field strengths. Likewise, studies with low-sensitivity nuclei become possible. Increased sensitivity may be traded off for shorter scanner time or higher spatial resolution (smaller volumes may be explored).

Magnetic Resonance Spectroscopy Applied to Brain Biochemistry

Proton MRS

MRS of the hydrogen nucleus or proton allows detection of more than a dozen metabolites involved in different aspects of intermediary metabolism. Some of the main ones are *N*-acetyl-aspartate (NAA), glutamate, glutamine, γ-aminobutyric acid (GABA), glutathione, creatine, phosphocreatine (PCr), choline (Cho), phosphocholine (PCh), glycerophosphocholine (GPC), glucose, taurine, inositol, and lactate.

Here we briefly review the spectral characteristics as well as the physiological significance of some of the observed metabolic pools. Although NAA is the most prominent compound in the brain proton spectrum, there is still no consensus concerning its function. Because it is mainly found in neurons and synthesized in the mitochondria, it is considered a marker of viable neurons. Hypotheses regarding its possible function include roles in osmotic regulation and synthesis of the neurotransmitter acetylcholine. Creatine and PCr appear in the proton spectrum as a single resonance peak (Cr; Figure 5–1) that is often used as a concentration reference standard. Both are involved in energy metabolism; creatine is formed after high-energy PCr has transferred its orthophosphate moiety to ADP to regenerate ATP, thus maintaining the ATP pool with its energy potential. That the Cr resonance peak is often used as a reference concentration standard reflects the fact that the total concentration of creatine and PCr is similar in many brain regions, although it is slightly higher in the cerebral cortex than in white matter. Choline-containing compounds involved in membrane metabolism—mainly PCh and GPC—give rise to the Cho resonance peak. Most of the choline in the brain is incorporated into the membrane phospholipid phosphatidylcholine, which has a restricted range of motion and thus is largely invisible to in vivo MRS. Inositol is involved in second-messenger neurotransmission (via phosphatidylinositols), phospho-

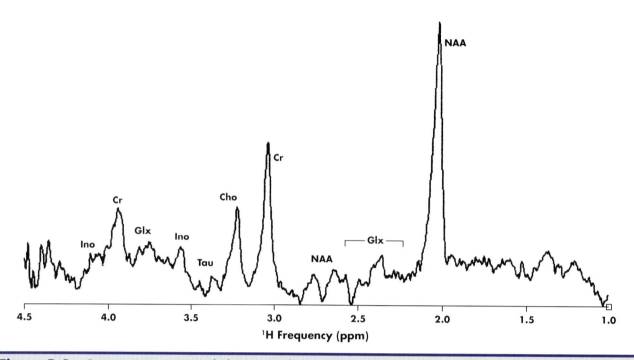

Figure 5–1. Proton spectrum recorded on a 4-tesla magnetic resonance scanner of brain tissue in vivo from a healthy 21-year-old man.

Point-resolved spectroscopy (PRESS) recording from a 6-mL volume localized in the motor cortex, right hemisphere; volume size=6 mL, echo time=23 msec, repetition time=3000 msec, 64 averages. Apodization with line broadening of 2.5 Hz applied. Abbreviations for peaks: Cho=choline compounds (choline, phosphocholine, glycerophosphocholine); Cr=creatine and phosphocreatine; Glx=spectral region of peaks for glutamate, glutamine, and GABA; Ino=myoinositol; NAA=*N*-acetyl-aspartate; Tau=taurine.

lipid metabolism, and osmotic equilibrium maintenance.

Phosphorus MRS

^{31}P MRS allows detection of compounds that play a key role in energy metabolism and membrane phospholipid metabolism. The resonance peaks of the nucleoside phosphates ATP and ADP and of NADPH present some overlap in the brain ^{31}P spectrum. ATP is the main contributor to the nucleoside triphosphate (NTP) peaks (Figure 5–2). The prominent PCr peak is often used as the chemical shift reference standard, set to zero ppm. The chemical shift of unbound inorganic phosphate (Pi) is dependent on pH and thus may be used to measure alterations in pH. Information on alterations in brain energy metabolism may be gained by measuring the relative levels of PCr, NTP, and Pi. The brain resonance peak of phosphomonoester (PME) arises primarily from the phospholipid precursors phosphoethanolamine and PCh, as well as from sugar

phosphates. The phosphodiester (PDE) resonance peak has a broad component (arising from membrane bilayers) and a narrow component (derived from the phospholipid catabolites GPC and glycerophosphoethanolamine).

Fluorine MRS

Except for trace amounts in bone and teeth, the body contains no endogenous fluorine. However, several medications have one or more fluorine (^{19}F) atoms in their active structure. When a fluorinated drug is administered exogenously, ^{19}F acts as a natural, nonradioactive, stable label detectable by MRS. There is no endogenous background signal. Quantitative analysis of the fluorine signal can yield brain concentrations of the medication in question, expectedly more closely related to the treatment and side effects of the drug than are plasma concentrations. Pharmacokinetics can thus be assessed in the target tissue as opposed to plasma.

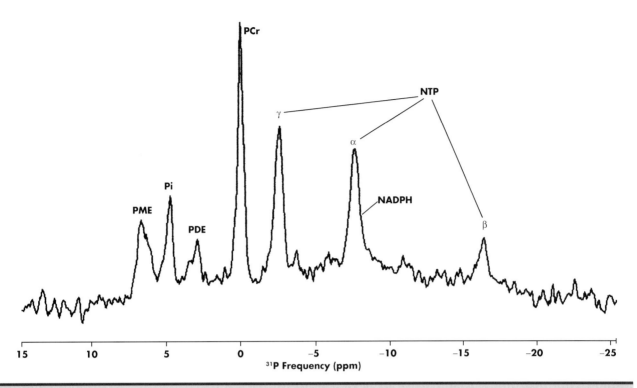

Figure 5–2. Phosphorus spectrum recorded on a 4-tesla magnetic resonance scanner of brain tissue in vivo from a healthy 33-year-old woman.
Spin-echo recording from an axial slice localized at the level of the corpus callosum; slice thickness=25 mm, field of view=240×240 mm, echo-time=18 msec, repetition time=2000 msec, 64 averages. Apodization with line broadening of 10 Hz applied. Abbreviations for peaks: α=alpha-NTP; β=beta-NTP; γ=gamma-NTP; NADPH= nicotinamide adenine dinucleotide phosphate; NTP= nucleoside triphosphate; PCr=phosphocreatine; PDE= phosphodiester; Pi=inorganic phosphate; PME=phosphomonoester.

Carbon-13 MRS

Although carbon is found in the body in abundance, its most plentiful isotope, ^{12}C, does not have a magnetic moment and is thus not detectable by MRS. The MRS-detectable nucleus ^{13}C has a natural abundance of 1.1%. Like ^{19}F, ^{13}C MRS has a low endogenous background signal, but in this case the low background signal is due to ^{13}C's low natural abundance combined with a low sensitivity. The low background allows for tracer studies: following administration of a compound enriched with ^{13}C (by organic synthesis of a compound in which the ^{12}C atoms at a particular position are replaced by ^{13}C), the ^{13}C signal from the compound will dominate the in vivo spectrum. Because naturally occurring metabolites can be labeled in this way, ^{13}C MRS provides a means of investigating the kinetics of intermediary metabolism. A main line of investigation with the ^{13}C MRS method involves tracing the appearance of breakdown products of glucose labeled with ^{13}C in various positions. Glucose is the main energetic substrate for the brain, and it is rapidly metabolized by the brain for pro-

duction of ATP via oxidative metabolism. The carbon backbone of glucose is not wasted, but is rapidly used to build the essential neurotransmitters glutamate and glutamine. In particular, the rate of glutamate synthesis from the moieties of glucose breakdown may thus be estimated by ^{13}C MRS methods. This rate is related to brain glutamatergic activity, which may be altered in psychiatric disorders. Treatment effects on glutamatergic activity may be observed by this method.

Lithium MRS

Lithium is a monovalent cation naturally found in trace amounts in biological systems; it occupies the same column as sodium in the periodic table of the elements and (with an electron shell smaller than that of sodium) is known to interact with sodium channels. When lithium is used as a mood stabilizer, particularly in bipolar disorder, tissue levels increase to MRS-detectable levels. Because therapeutic serum levels are in the range of 1 millimole per liter, brain lithium levels may be detected and quantified with relative ease.

Contributions of Magnetic Resonance Methods to Clinical Neuropsychiatric Research

In this section we review some of the clinical areas in which MRS has made relevant contributions. This gives the background for the possible future developments in clinical MR applied to psychiatry.

Cognitive Disorders

Neurodegeneration associated with dementia may be assessed from NAA levels in the hippocampus, as demonstrated in early postmortem studies of Alzheimer's disease and as suggested by in vivo studies of dementia of the Alzheimer's type. A current limitation in Alzheimer's disease management is the inability to obtain a definitive diagnosis before death and without postmortem chemical analysis of the brain tissue for presence of plaques and tangles. Thus, MRS measurement of NAA levels in regions of the brain related to memory and executive function—the parahippocampal gyrus, the temporal and frontal lobes—is used in explorations of cognitive disorders.

Schizophrenia

MRS research in schizophrenia has increased nearly exponentially in the past dozen years or so. Two major findings have emerged from the literature. The first is decreased PME and increased PDE in the frontal lobe, as determined by ^{31}P MRS. Overall decreased brain PDE in schizophrenia patients relative to healthy control subjects has also been reported. The second major finding is focal decreases in NAA in the frontal and temporal lobes in both neuroleptic-naive and treated patients with schizophrenia.

Affective Illness

Major Depression

Decreased levels of both beta-NTP and total NTP have been found in the basal ganglia and in the frontal lobes bilaterally with ^{31}P MRS. These results are surprising, given that cerebral ATP levels are expected to be maintained at the expense of PCr. However, these data are consistent with findings in disorders associated with sustained cerebral hypometabolism.

Increases as well as decreases in the intensity of the Cho resonance peak have been observed in depressed populations with ^{1}H MRS. Variations in findings may be attributable to differences in the brain regions studied, in MRS recording conditions, or in characteristics of the study population. However, baseline estimates of Cho signal intensity, as well as change with treatment, have been shown to correlate with clinical response.

Depressed subjects have been reported to have decreased myoinositol levels in the right frontal lobe, detected via ^{1}H MRS, compared with age- and gender-matched healthy comparison subjects. This finding suggests the possibility that the phosphatidylinositol second-messenger system may be reduced in depression.

Occipital lobe GABA levels have been reported to be dramatically reduced, by more than 50%, in patients with major depression. This finding is in line with the GABA hypothesis of mood disorders, which posits that low GABA function is an inherited biological marker of vulnerability for development of mood disorders. Reduced glutamate levels in the anterior cingulate have also been reported in subjects with major depression. Both glutamate and N-methyl-D-aspartate receptors have been implicated in the pathophysiology of depression. Should these findings be replicated, they will enhance our understanding of the biochemical basis of this serious illness and could well lead to new treatment strategies.

Bipolar Disorder

A major finding in a comprehensive series of studies indicates that frontal lobe PME levels determined by ^{31}P MRS vary with mood state. In addition, the intensity of the Cho and myoinositol resonance of ^{1}H MRS has been shown to be altered in bipolar patients. These results may be related to the action of lithium, which inhibits Cho transport across membranes and alters myoinositol metabolism. Alternatively, these findings may be closely related to PME variations, considering that ^{31}P PME signals derive primarily from PCh and phosphoethanolamine and that ^{1}H MRS choline signals are derived from PCh and GPC.

Anxiety Disorders

Panic Disorder

The ability to assess lactate levels with ^{1}H MRS has allowed exploration of lactate's role in the brain in panic attacks. Intravenous infusion of sodium lactate is known to induce panic attacks in most patients with panic disorder. A ^{1}H MRS finding is that lactate-induced panic is associated with increased and prolonged elevations in brain lactate relative to values observed in comparison subjects. Similar findings have been observed following controlled hyperventilation in panic patients, suggesting that these individuals may have increased sensitivity to hypocapnia.

Abnormalities of phosphorous metabolism in panic disorder are also suggested by a ^{31}P MRS study that reported a significant asymmetry (left > right) of PCr concentration in the frontal lobes of patients with panic disorder compared with healthy control subjects (Shioiri et al. 1996). This finding is in line with earlier studies with SPECT and electroencephalography (EEG), which also noted frontal lobe right–left asymmetries in patients with panic disorder.

Another ^{1}H MRS study demonstrating a 22% reduction in total occipital cortex GABA concentration (GABA plus homocarnosine) in patients with panic disorder compared with control subjects (Goddard et al. 2001) provided preliminary evidence that reduction in GABA levels might contribute to the pathophysiology of panic disorder.

Obsessive-Compulsive Disorder

Results from ^{1}H MRS studies demonstrating decreased levels of NAA in the striatum and the anterior cingulate of obsessive-compulsive disorder (OCD) patients suggest reduced neuronal density in this region of the brain, although no significant difference in caudate volumes between groups has been found. These findings remain controversial, given that other studies have revealed no differences in NAA levels in the lenticular nuclei between OCD and healthy subjects. PET studies have noted that the basal ganglia may play an important role in mediating mechanisms of action for effective treatments in persons with OCD. Thus, MRS findings of decreased NAA levels in OCD patients are in line with the hypothesis that orbitofrontal–subcortical circuit function mediates the symptomatic expression of OCD.

Treatment-naive children and adolescents with OCD were found to have increased composite Glx (glutamate, glutamine, and GABA) resonance peaks in the ^{1}H MRS spectrum from the caudate nucleus region in comparison with healthy control subjects (Rosenberg et al. 2000). Because the Glx resonance in the caudate region is presumed to derive primarily from glutamate, these findings suggest a relationship between OCD and anomalies in glutamatergic function in the caudate. The composite Glx resonance was found to decrease significantly with paroxetine treatment in several studies (Moore et al. 1998; Rosenberg et al. 2000). In addition, decreases in caudate glutamatergic concentrations were found to correlate with decreases in OCD symptom severity (Rosenberg et al. 2000). These results are consistent with those of a PET study in adult OCD subjects (Saxena et al. 1999), in which treatment produced a significant decrease in glucose metabolism in the orbitofrontal cortex and right caudate.

Posttraumatic Stress Disorder

^{1}H MRS studies of NAA levels in the medial temporal lobes in patients with posttraumatic stress disorder (PTSD) reveal significantly lower NAA in the right temporal lobe relative to the left temporal lobe (Freeman et al. 1998). These findings suggest lateralized decreases in neuronal density in medial temporal lobes in PTSD subjects. This change might be due, in part, to the initial emotional stress and subsequent high blood cortisol levels. These results are also in line with those of MRI volumetric studies documenting decreases on the order of 8% in right hippocampal volumes of PTSD patients relative to healthy comparison subjects (Bremner et al. 1995).

Anterior cingulate NAA levels measured via ^{1}H MRS in children and adolescents with PTSD were found to be significantly decreased in comparison with healthy subjects (De Bellis et al. 2000). The results of this study suggest that neuronal pathology in the anterior cingulate may mediate symptoms in childhood PTSD.

Substance Abuse Disorders

Alcohol Abuse

Ethyl alcohol can be detected with ^{1}H MRS, and subjective reports of intoxication have been shown to parallel ^{1}H MRS measurement of brain alcohol levels. Studies with ^{1}H MRS have suggested that alcohol tolerance may be determined by differences in the interaction of ethanol with brain membranes, possibly reflecting decreased membrane fluidity.

The neurochemical effects of medications used to treat alcoholism have been explored with ^{1}H MRS in healthy volunteer subjects. Acamprosate, which has been found to be useful in maintaining abstinence following alcohol withdrawal in chronic alcoholism, was shown to decrease brain ^{1}H MR spectral intensities in regions in which glutamate and NAA are the main signal contributors, at time points associated with maximum plasmatic concentration (Bolo et al. 1998). These results are consistent with a central glutamatergic action of acamprosate, which has been demonstrated by microdialysis measurements taken in the nucleus accumbens of rats (Dahchour et al. 1998). Hypotheses for mechanisms of action of medication treatments can thus be explored with ^{1}H MRS methods.

Cocaine and Polydrug Abuse

Cocaine users have been reported to show decreased NAA in the frontal cortex and increased myoinositol in frontal gray and white matter (Chang et al. 1997). Decreased levels of NAA in the left thalamus have been found in chronic cocaine abusers compared with healthy comparison subjects (Li et al. 1999). An assessment of the intensity of basal ganglia ^{1}H MRS metabolite resonances following acute administration of cocaine in healthy subjects revealed increased levels of Cho and NAA in the basal ganglia, possibly consistent with cell swelling (Christensen et al. 2000).

In addition, altered brain phospholipid metabolites in cocaine-dependent polysubstance abusers have been demonstrated by ^{31}P MRS (MacKay et al. 1993). Polysubstance (cocaine and heroin)–abusing men had increased PME and decreased ATP levels compared with healthy comparison subjects (Christensen et al. 1996). Cerebral PME and PDE levels are increased and PCr level is decreased in opiate-dependent polydrug abusers (Kaufman et al. 1999).

Current Trends in Clinical Psychiatric Magnetic Resonance

Diagnosis

In pathological processes characterized by gross structural changes, such as the neurodegenerative dementias, large MRS changes accompany the changes that are observable by MRI. The added diagnostic value of the MRS information is limited in such disorders, given that massive neuronal cell death will already be obvious from other neuroimaging modalities. MRS studies are expected to be most valuable when they are able to discern small biochemical changes undetectable by other modalities. For Alzheimer's disease, detection of

decreases in NAA levels in the parahippocampal gyrus offers potential for early detection of loss of viable neurons indicative of a neurodegenerative process.

The diagnostic value of MRS combined with other MR methods has been well demonstrated in the evaluation of epilepsy. In unilateral mesial temporal lobe epilepsy, the combined measurement of NAA level and T2 relaxation time was able to classify hippocampus anomalies (Namer et al. 1999). Low NAA and elevated T2 values corresponded to abnormalities observed in sclerotic ipsilateral hippocampus, whereas low NAA with slightly elevated or normal T2 values was found contralaterally. Furthermore, the combined measurement was shown to correlate with both clinical severity and memory performance. Left hippocampal injury evaluated by NAA levels and by T2 relaxation time measurements correlated with verbal memory scores, and right hippocampal injury correlated with visual memory scores. The value of the combined MRS–MR examination in presurgical evaluation of patients lies in the ability to detect changes in the contralateral hippocampus that present no anomalies in other neuroimaging modalities.

Treatment Planning

Several studies that used quantitative MRS methods to determine steady-state brain concentrations of the selective serotonin reuptake inhibitors (SSRIs) fluvoxamine and fluoxetine yielded similar results (Bolo et al. 2000; Renshaw et al. 1992; Strauss et al. 1997). This convergence of results is promising for the goal of ^{19}F MRS to attain clinical usefulness as an aid in elucidating treatment and side effects. The differences in brain-to-serum ratios of fluvoxamine in major depressive disorder versus obsessive-compulsive disorder found by ^{19}F MRS in separate studies (Bolo et al. 2000; Strauss et al. 1997) indicate that ^{19}F MRS may be used to characterize metabolic profile responses to the SSRIs in different patient populations. Individual pharmacokinetic profiles of SSRIs may prove useful to the clinician for dosage and treatment planning.

Future Directions

Psychotropic Drug Development

MRS may be performed in conjunction with administration to healthy volunteers of a medication with a known treatment effect. Baseline metabolic profiles obtained via MRS may be compared with postadministration profiles. The changes observed in the brain spectrum after administration—which hypothetically should be related to action of the medication—may be used to explore the mechanism of action of the medication. The MRS recording, derived from a volume of interest inside the brain, provides an objective measurement of the treatment's biochemical effects in the central nervous system (CNS). In the case where a drug has well-characterized efficacy or behavioral effects in a given patient population, the additional information provided by the MRS recordings should help to elucidate the links between the drug's structure, pharmacology, and biochemistry and its treatment effect. Medications could thus be described by their in vivo metabolic profiles. With MRS, the metabolic effect is measured directly in the target organ. Further development of research along these lines could lead to new target profiles that would be based on in vivo CNS biochemical drug effects as assessed by MRS methods.

Just as knowledge is gained through assessment of the neurochemical dynamics associated with medications with established treatment efficacy records, the pharmacological challenge method applied with MRS should likewise open new pathways for exploring underlying mechanisms of psychiatric disorders. Compounds whose effects reversibly simulate one or several aspects of a behavioral symptom associated with a disorder can be administered under well-controlled conditions to healthy volunteers. In vivo assessment of CNS metabolites via MRS can track the link between the dynamics both of behavior and of the underlying neurochemistry. Because these methods are founded on rigorous experimental control of very specific reversible effects, they have the potential to yield the highly reliable and reproducible results required for evaluation of new treatments.

The same MRS methodology can thus be extended to the development of new compounds. In the realm of treatments for psychiatric disorders, the behavioral target is often a particular neurotransmitter system. The MRS recording in vivo may provide a means to determine whether the newly developed compound is acting upon that system in the expected way. In characterizing the CNS effects of new compounds under development, studies that simultaneously record CNS chemistry by MRS and behavioral effects by interactive neurocognitive testing should be of great value. The correlation between behavioral scores and neurochemical dynamics needs to be further explored. Research that establishes links between specific behavioral effects and neurochemical effects assessed by MRS should provide a powerful means of evaluating the potential treatment efficacy of new compounds. As with early diagnosis of neurodegenerative diseases, the added value of MRS in psychopharmacology resides in its potential to detect chemical changes before massive behavioral effects are present or when behavioral testing yields contradictory or unreliable results. In this sense, with further development of well-designed experimental methods, MRS has the potential to yield surrogate markers for many psychiatric disorders and their treatment effects. The pharmacological challenge method provides an example of how such a marker would work: the MRS-observed change induced by the pharmacological challenge should be reversed or blocked by the new treatment.

The particular ability of ^{13}C MRS to track glutamatergic and glutaminergic neurotransmitter dynamics with drug administration should lead to more rapid development of treatments for the disorders involving these pathways. The glutamatergic neurotransmitter system has been implicated in schizophrenia, mood disorders, and anxiety disorders; thus, it may become an immediate candidate as a new pharmacological target for these disorders. ^{13}C MRS can help explore the CNS effects of such novel treatment strategies.

Evaluation of Potential Treatment Efficacy

MRS can be used to evaluate the potential efficacy of a treatment by characterizing the neurochemical effects of the treatment in specific areas of the brain. Levels of NAA in the hippocampus have been shown to correlate with memory function. In the same way that restored NAA levels indicate restored function in epilepsy or dementias, other MRS markers in specific areas may provide a means of evaluating whether treatments are likely to be efficacious. Such markers could have value for early identification of likely responders and nonresponders to a given medication. For example, further investigations by MRS confirming the link between the neurotransmitter GABA and anxiety could lead to evaluation of panic disorder treatments by their ability to restore GABA levels. Glutamate levels or glutamate synthesis rates observed in the prefrontal cortex by ^{13}C MRS could be good candidates to help evaluate treatment potential in mood, anxiety, or psychosis-related disorders.

Conclusions

The ability of MRS to nonsurgically extract specific biochemical information from localized regions inside the body without the use of either radioactively labeled tracers (in contrast to PET or SPECT, for example) or high-energy electromagnetic radiation (in contrast to X-ray tomography, for example) makes it a unique and powerful tool for the clinical psychiatrist. Although MRS holds great potential for facilitating the processes of diagnosis (as is the case for lateralization in focal epilepsies) and of treatment planning, its actual clinical use is as yet limited, because it is still a relatively new technology in the psychiatric clinical arena. However, MRS has proven itself invaluable in clinical research for a variety of psychiatric disorders, including cognitive disorders, schizophrenia, affective and anxiety disorders, and substance abuse disorders. MRS yields markers of biochemical processes related to the pathophysiology of psychiatric disorders. Measurements of regional levels of NAA (indicating viable neuron density) are of value in examining neurodegenerative as well as reversible disease processes that lead to various types of cognitive disorders. MRS allows exploration of various aspects of regional energetic metabolism, membrane metabolism, and second-messenger metabolism through its ability to evaluate levels of relevant metabolic pools in schizophrenia or in mood or substance abuse disorders. MRS can be used to assess the activity of specific neurotransmitter pathways (e.g., the GABA or glutamatergic pathways) in anxiety or other psychiatric disorders. Some drugs may be assayed via MRS, with concentrations measured in the target organ in vivo, thus allowing tissue pharmacokinetic and pharmacodynamic studies to be performed on both short (hours to days) and longer (weeks to months to years) time scales. Because of its versatility, MRS has the potential to greatly accelerate the development of new treatments of psychiatric disorders by helping to assess the CNS effects of novel treatments, by allowing the testing of novel mechanistic hypotheses of drug actions, and by aiding in evaluating treatment efficacy of novel compounds or treatment strategies.

References

Bolo NR, Rode Y, Nedelec J, et al: Brain pharmacokinetics and tissue distribution in vivo of fluvoxamine and fluoxetine by fluorine magnetic resonance spectroscopy. Neuropsychopharmacology 23:428–438, 2000

Bolo NR, Nedelec JF, Muzet M, et al: Central effects of acamprosate: part 2. Acamprosate modifies the brain in-vivo proton magnetic resonance spectrum in healthy young male volunteers. Psychiatry Res 82:115–127, 1998

Chang L, Mehringer CM, Ernst T, et al: Neurochemical alterations in asymptomatic abstinent cocaine users: a proton magnetic resonance spectroscopy study. Biol Psychiatry 42:1105–1114, 1997

Christensen JD, Kaufman MJ, Levin JM, et al: Abnormal cerebral metabolism in polydrug abusers during early withdrawal: a 31P MR spectroscopy study. Magn Reson Med 35:658–663, 1996

Christensen JD, Kaufman MJ, Frederick B, et al: Proton magnetic resonance spectroscopy of human basal ganglia: response to cocaine administration. Biol Psychiatry 48:685–692, 2000

Dahchour A, De Witte P, Bolo NR, et al: Central effects of acamprosate: part 1. Acamprosate blocks the glutamate increase in the nucleus accumbens microdialysate in ethanol withdrawn rats. Psychiatry Res 82:107–114, 1998

Bremner JD, Randall P, Scott TM, et al: MRI-based measurement of hippocampal volume in patients with combat-related posttraumatic stress disorder. Am J Psychiatry 152:973–981, 1995

De Bellis MD, Keshavan MS, Spencer S, et al: N-Acetylaspartate concentration in the anterior cingulate of maltreated children and adolescents with PTSD. Am J Psychiatry 157:1175–1177, 2000

Freeman TW, Cardwell D, Karson CN, et al: In vivo proton magnetic resonance spectroscopy of the medial temporal lobes of subjects with combat-related posttraumatic stress disorder. Magn Reson Med 40:66–71, 1998

Goddard AW, Mason GF, Almai A, et al: Reductions in occipital cortex GABA levels in panic disorder detected with 1H-magnetic resonance spectroscopy. Arch Gen Psychiatry 58:556–561, 2001

Kaufman MJ, Pollack MH, Villafuerte RA, et al: Cerebral phosphorus metabolite abnormalities in opiate-dependent polydrug abusers in methadone maintenance. Psychiatry Res 90:143–152, 1999

Li SI, Wang Y, Pankiewicz I, et al: Neurochemical adaptation to cocaine abuse: reduction of N-acetyl aspartate in thalamus of human cocaine abusers. Biol Psychiatry 45:1481–1487, 1999

MacKay S, Meyerhoff DI, Dillon WP, et al: Alteration of brain phospholipid metabolites in cocaine-dependent polysubstance abusers. Biol Psychiatry 34:261–264, 1993

Moore GJ, MacMaster FP, Stewart C, et al: Case study: caudate glutamatergic changes with paroxetine therapy for pediatric obsessive-compulsive disorder. J Am Acad Child Adolesc Psychiatry 37:663–667, 1998

Namer IJ, Bolo NR, Sellal F, et al: Combination of hippocampal N-acetyl-aspartate and T2 relaxation time measurements for the evaluation of temporal lobe epilepsy. Correlation with clinical severity and memory performance. Epilepsia 40:1424–1432, 1999

Renshaw PF, Guimaraes AR, Fava M, et al: Accumulation of fluoxetine and norfluoxetine in human brain during therapeutic administration. Am J Psychiatry 149:1592–1594, 1992

Rosenberg DR, MacMaster FP, Keshavall MS, et al: Decrease in caudate glutamatergic concentrations in pediatric obsessive-compulsive disorder patients taking paroxetine. J Am Acad Child Adolesc Psychiatry 39:1096–1103, 2000

Saxena S, Brody AL, Maidment KM, et al: Localized orbitofrontal and subcortical metabolic changes and predictors of response to paroxetine treatment in obsessive-compulsive disorder. Neuropsychopharmacology 21:683–693, 1999

Shioiri T, Kato T, Murashita J, et al: High-energy phosphate metabolism in the frontal lobes of patients with panic disorder detected by phase-encoded 31P MRS. Biol Psychiatry 40:785–793, 1996

Slichter C: Principles of Magnetic Resonance, 3rd Edition, Vol 1. New York, Springer-Verlag, 1996

Strauss WL, Layton ME, Hayes CE, et al: 19F magnetic resonance spectroscopy investigation in vivo of acute and steady-state brain fluvoxamine levels in obsessive-compulsive disorder. Am J Psychiatry 154:516–522, 1997

Suggested Readings

Dager SR, Friedman SD, Heide A, et al: Two-dimensional proton echo-planar spectroscopic imaging of brain metabolic changes during lactate-induced panic. Arch Gen Psychiatry 56:70–77, 1999

Kato T, Inubushi T, Kato N: Magnetic resonance spectroscopy in affective disorders. J Neuropsychiatry Clin Neurosci 10: 133–147, 1998

Komoroski RA: Applications of (7)Li NMR in biomedicine. Magn Reson Imaging 18:103–116, 2000

Pouwels PJ, Frahm J: Regional metabolite concentrations in human brain as determined by quantitative localized proton MRS. Magn Reson Med 39:53–60, 1998

Soares JC, Boada F, Keshavan MS: Brain lithium measurements with (7)Li magnetic resonance spectroscopy (MRS): a literature review. Eur Neuropsychopharmacol 10:151–158, 2000

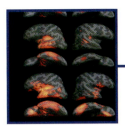

6

Electroencephalography, Event-Related Potentials, and Magnetoencephalography

Gina R. Kuperberg, M.D., Ph.D.

In this chapter I discuss the use of electroencephalography, event-related potentials, and magnetoencephalography in psychiatry. Of these three measures, electroencephalography is the only one that is currently used in standard psychiatric clinical practice, and even here, its main use is to exclude certain neurological disorders in the differential diagnosis of psychiatric disorders. Event-related potentials and magnetoencephalography currently have no direct clinical applications in psychiatry. Nonetheless, they are both the focus of intense research interest. This is because these methods, of all the noninvasive neuroimaging techniques, provide the most direct measure of neurocognitive function with the greatest temporal resolution.

The main aim of this chapter is to serve as in introduction to each of these techniques. Each section begins with a description of how the relevant signals are extracted, followed by a summary of some of the technique's applications in psychiatric clinical practice or research.

The Electroencephalogram

Generation of Signal

Conventional Electroencephalography

If a pair of electrodes is attached to the surface of the scalp and connected to an amplifier, the output of the amplifier shows a variation in voltage over time. This pattern of voltage variation is known as the electroencephalogram (EEG). The amplitude of the normal EEG varies between approximately −100 and +100 microvolts, and its frequency ranges to 40 Hertz (Hz) or more. Figure 6–1 shows a standard placement of electrodes over the scalp.

The EEG signal does not arise from individual action potentials; rather, it derives from the extracellular current flow that is associated with excitatory postsynaptic potentials (EPSPs) and inhibitory postsynaptic potentials (IPSPs). These current flows are of much lower voltage than action potentials. They are, however, distributed across a large surface area of membrane and are of longer durations than action potentials, allowing summation. Even with summation, however, the fields produced by individual neurons are much too weak to be detected by the EEG at the surface of the scalp. In order to generate externally detectable signals, the neurons within a volume of tissue must be aligned, and their synaptic current flows must be correlated in time. Of all the neurons in the human brain, the cortical pyramidal cells are particularly well suited to generate externally observable electric fields. This is because of their elongated apical dendrites, which are systematically aligned in a columnar fashion, perpendicular to the cortical sheet.

Although much of the amplitude of the brain electrical activity derives from cortical neurons underlying the scalp electrodes, the synchronicity of the recorded activity is largely regulated by subcortical sites. For example, pacemaker neurons within the thalamus normally oscillate synchronously, producing an alpha rhythm that characterizes the EEG of an awake healthy person at rest. Such synchrony is reduced by arousal. Desynchronization of electrical activity is thought to be mediated by afferent projections from the reticular formation and basal forebrain. These effects may be modulated by noradrenergic, cholinergic, and γ-aminobutyric acid (GABA)ergic neuronal systems. Brain electrical frequencies are generally reported in the delta (0–4 Hz), theta (4–8 Hz), alpha (8–13 Hz), and beta (>13 Hz) bands. Figure 6–2 shows examples of alpha and beta activity.

Quantitative Electroencephalography

EEGs have traditionally been evaluated by visual inspection of paper tracings. To quantify measurements of the frequency content of the EEG, the digitized signal can be recorded on magnetic or optical media. The quantitative EEG (qEEG) provides information that cannot reliably be extracted from visual inspection of the EEG. It has been argued that such qEEG estimates improve intra- and interrater reliability and yield reproducible estimates that can be compared over time

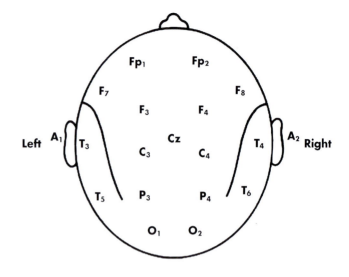

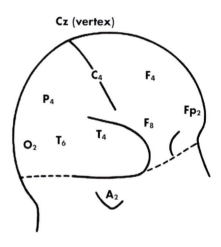

Figure 6–1. Standard placement of EEG recording electrodes at the top and sides of the head. Abbreviations for electrode placements: A = auricle; C = central; Cz = vertex; F = frontal; Fp = frontal pole; O = occipital; P = parietal; T = temporal. The multiple electrode placements overlying a given area (e.g., temporal) are indicated by numerical subscripts. Placement C_4 overlies the region of the central sulcus. *Source.* Reprinted from Kandel ER, Schwartz JH, Jessell TM (eds.): *Principles of Neural Science,* 3rd Edition. New York, McGraw-Hill, 1991, p. 779. Copyright 1991, The McGraw-Hill Companies. Used with permission.

in single individuals. Once digital data are recorded, they can be transformed through use of the Fourier transformation algorithm from the domain of "amplitude versus frequency" to a domain of "power versus frequency." The qEEG gives rise to a number of different measures. For example, *absolute power* is a measure of the intensity of energy measured in microvolts

Left

Frontal

Beta

Temporal

Occipital

Right

Frontal

Occipital

Alpha

1 sec

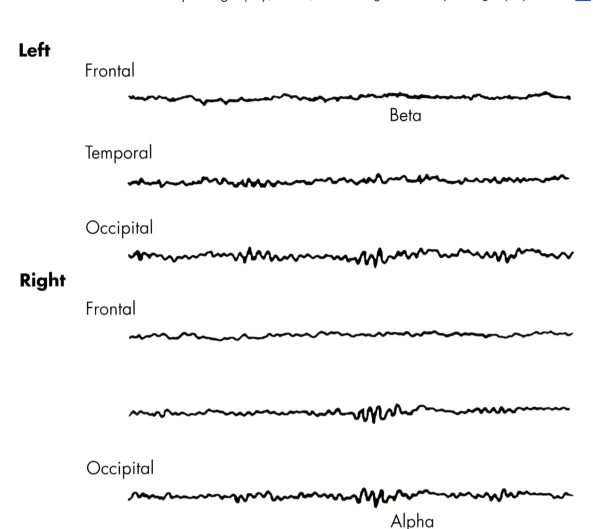

Figure 6–2.　Electroencephalogram (EEG) recorded in a human subject at rest from the scalp surface at various points over the left and right hemispheres.

Three pairs of EEG electrodes are positioned so as to overlie the frontal, temporal, and occipital lobes. Beta activity—the EEG activity with the highest frequency and lowest amplitude—is recorded over the frontal lobes. Alpha activity—a signature of a brain in a relaxed and wakeful state—is recorded in the occipital and temporal lobes. The presence of alpha activity in the occipital lobe suggests that the subject's eyes were closed.

Source.　Reprinted from Kandel ER, Schwartz JH, Jessell TM (eds.): *Principles of Neural Science*, 3rd Edition. New York, McGraw-Hill, 1991, p. 778. Copyright 1991, The McGraw-Hill Companies. Used with permission.

squared and calculated in a series of frequency bands (the *power spectrum*) for approximately 25 seconds. Another important measure is *coherence*—a measure of the *phase consistency* of two signals (i.e., the extent to which EEG signals from different brain regions have frequency components that are time-locked to each other). Coherence varies between 0 and 1 and is analogous to a correlation coefficient of the signal between two brain areas. It is thought to reflect the degree of functional connectivity between brain regions, although its functional physiological significance remains unclear.

Clinical Use in Psychiatric Practice

When electroencephalography was first introduced by Hans Berger in 1929, the hope was that it would directly aid the diagnosis of the major mental disorders—schizophrenia, depression, and anxiety. This hope has long since been abandoned. Nonetheless, the EEG remains a valuable part of psychiatric clinical practice. It is mainly helpful in the diagnosis of neurological disorders—such as delirium, dementia, and epilepsy—that must often be ruled out in the differential diagnosis of many "nonorganic" psychiatric disorders.

Although the EEG does not play a direct role in the diagnosis of psychiatric disorders, the EEGs in such disorders often do show abnormal (although nonspecific) features. In the following sections, I summarize some characteristic features of the EEG in dementia, delirium, schizophrenia, and other psychiatric disorders.

Dementias

In general, the EEG in patients with dementia is characterized by relatively low-frequency rhythms with an increase in the amount of delta and theta waves and a relative decrease in the amount of high-frequency beta activity. In addition, the alpha rhythm is slowed, and in some individuals its normal suppression to eye opening is not observed. These features may be particularly helpful in distinguishing dementia from depression in elderly persons.

It is thought that at least half of the individuals with minimal impairment on the Mini-Mental State Examination show some EEG abnormalities. It has therefore been suggested that the EEG may aid the diagnosis of dementia at an early stage in the disease course. Moreover, increased slow activity is correlated with cognitive impairment and measures of clinical severity in Alzheimer's disease. qEEG studies in dementia are consistent with conventional EEG findings, confirming increased delta and/or theta power.

Although the etiology of dementia cannot be determined by use of the EEG alone, certain types of dementia are characterized by particular EEG features. For example, focal EEG abnormalities are more common in vascular dementias (although not in diffuse white matter ischemic disease [Binswanger's disease]) than in primary degenerative dementias. In frontotemporal dementias such as Pick's disease, the posterior dominant background rhythm is relatively well preserved, whereas increases in slow waves are less pronounced and, when they occur, tend to be distributed anteriorly. In Creutzfeldt-Jakob disease, the EEG is characterized by frontally distributed triphasic waves and paroxysmal epileptiform discharges.

Delirium

The hallmark of the EEG in delirium is a slowing of the background rhythm. The exception to this is delirium tremens, in which the EEG is characterized by fast rhythms. The appearance of generalized slow-wave activity during a delirium often parallels the severity and time course of alternations in consciousness. In addition to increased slowing, other specific EEG patterns

are associated with particular metabolic encephalopathies. For example, frontal triphasic waves at a frequency of 2 or 3 per second are particularly characteristic of a hepatic encephalopathy and may also occur in patients with chronic renal failure.

Schizophrenia

There are no EEG changes that are specific to schizophrenia. Nonetheless, across a large number of studies, there is some consensus that patients with schizophrenia show a high incidence of EEG abnormalities, including increased delta and theta rhythms. Evaluation of the EEG in schizophrenia is complicated by the heterogeneity of the disorder itself and by the effects of medication. Indeed, the incidence of EEG abnormalities may be particularly high in patients taking atypical antipsychotic drugs such as clozapine and olanzapine.

Other Psychiatric Disorders

The incidence of abnormal EEG findings in mood disorders is thought to range from 20%–40%. Small sharp spikes and paroxysmal events have been described, and there are numerous reports of abnormal sleep patterns. Several studies have also suggested a high incidence of EEG abnormalities in anxiety disorders, including panic disorder and obsessive-compulsive disorder. There is no marked consistency across studies, however, in the precise patterns of abnormalities.

Event-Related Potentials

In the following subsections, I consider the issue of how an ERP component is defined and provide a brief overview of some of the better known ERP components that have been studied in psychiatric disorders.

Generation of Signal: Selective Averaging of EEG to Derive ERPs

Event-related potentials (ERPs) are voltage fluctuations, derived from the ongoing EEG, that are time-locked to specific sensory, motor, or cognitive events (Figure 6–3).

Suppose a stimulus is presented to a subject during EEG recording. Some of the voltage changes may be specifically related to the brain's response to that stimulus. In most cases, the voltage changes occurring within

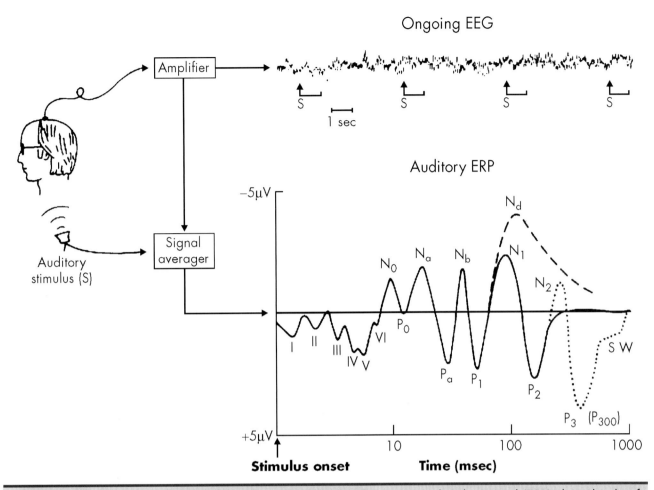

Figure 6–3.   Idealized waveform of computer-averaged auditory event-related potential (ERP) elicited to brief sound.

The ERP is generally too small to be detected in the ongoing electroencephalogram (EEG) *(top)* and requires computer averaging over many stimulus presentations to achieve adequate signal-to-noise ratios. The logarithmic time display allows visualization of the early brain-stem responses (waves I–VI), the midlatency components (N_0, P_0, N_a, P_a, and N_b), the "vertex potential" waves (P_1, N_1, and P_2), and the task-related endogenous components (N_d, N_2, P_3, and slow wave [SW]). S=auditory stimulus; μV=microvolts.

Source.   Reprinted from Hillyard SA, Kutas M: "Electrophysiology of Cognitive Processing." *Annual Review of Psychology* 34:33–61, 1983. Copyright 1983, Annual Reviews (www.annualreviews.org). Used with permission from *The Annual Review of Psychology,* Volume 34.

a particular *epoch* (time period) of EEG following an event are on the order of microvolts and are therefore too small to be reliably detected. The most common way of extracting the signal is therefore to record a number of EEG epochs, each time-locked to repetitions of the same event (or type of event), and to derive an average waveform. EEG activity that is not time-locked to the event will vary randomly across epochs; thus, this background activity will disappear to zero in the averaging procedure.

In early research, the term *evoked potentials* was used to describe these waveforms, because it was believed that the waveforms reflected brain activity that was directly "evoked" by the presentation of stimuli. Many of

these waveforms, however, are now thought to reflect processes that arise from the cognitive demands of the situation—hence the use of the more neutral term *event-related potentials.*

What Is an ERP "Component"?

Particular regions or temporal windows of the ERP waveform have been differentiated and labeled according to their polarity (positive [P] or negative [N]), their peak latency, and/or their ordinal position. These are called ERP components. ERP components have traditionally been classified as either *exogenous* (i.e., generally occurring within 200 msec of stimulus onset and determined by the physical nature of the eliciting stimulus) or *endogenous* (i.e., sensitive to changes in the state of the subject, the meaning of the stimulus, and/or the processing demands of the task). The question of what constitutes a distinct ERP component remains controversial. Most researchers define components on the basis of their polarity, their scalp distribution, their characteristic latency, and their sensitivity to experimental manipulations.

As a rule of thumb, differences in the polarity and/or scalp distribution are usually interpreted as reflecting the activity of distinct neuronal populations subserving qualitatively different neurocognitive processes. This is not necessarily the case, however, because a waveform observed on the surface of the scalp may result from the summation of electrical activity that may be generated by several different sources in the brain. Thus, an ERP peak may not necessarily reflect activity of a single neuronal generator but rather the combined activity of two (or more) generators maximally active before or after that peak, but with fields that summate to a maximum at the time of the peak.

Because ERPs are time-locked to specific events and their measurement does not require an overt response by the subject, they provide important information about the relative time course of cognitive events. Once again, however, it is difficult to extrapolate from the waveform seen at the surface of the scalp to the underlying neurocognitive process. For example, is it the timing of a peak itself that is more informative about cognitive processing, or is the timing of the peak's onset of most relevance? Does a peak appear when a particular cognitive process is complete? Or does it indicate that enough information has accumulated to cross threshold and trigger the onset of a cognitive operation?

Abnormalities in Specific ERP Components in Psychiatric Disorders

In this section, I briefly review four of the ERP components studied in psychiatric research—the contingent negative variation (CNV), the mismatch negativity (MMN), the P300, and the N400. I first provide a brief description of the paradigms that elicit each of these components, and then summarize studies that have examined these components in different psychiatric populations.

The Contingent Negative Variation

The CNV was first described by Walter and colleagues in 1964. In their original paradigm, a warning click was

presented, followed by a flashing light. The subject was required to press a button in response to the light. During the interval between the click and the light, a slow negative wave was observed that reached its peak at around the time of the light presentation—the CNV. The CNV was not evident when the click or the light was presented alone or when they were paired without the response requirement. Although it was originally described as an "expectancy" wave, more recently the CNV has been linked with the motor or goal-directed preparatory processes. Several studies have reported a reduced amplitude of the CNV in patients with schizophrenia and patients with depression. These findings have generally been interpreted fairly nonspecifically as reflecting abnormalities in attentional processes.

The Mismatch Negativity

At about 200 milliseconds (msec) following the presentation of auditory events that deviate in some way from the surrounding events, a negative component is observed—the N200 or N2. The difference waveform between the improbable events (signals) and the surrounding events (standards) is called the MMN. The MMN is observed in response to events that are improbable with respect to a number of factors, such as frequency and duration. It is seen in association with both attended and unattended events.

Several studies have reported that the MMN is reduced in patients with schizophrenia, particularly in response to events that are deviant in duration. A reduced MMN has been reported in both medicated and unmedicated patients as well as in unaffected first-degree relatives of patients. Functional magnetic resonance imaging (fMRI) findings suggest that patients with schizophrenia show abnormally reduced activity of the superior temporal cortex in association with mismatch events. It has been hypothesized that the reduced MMN in patients with schizophrenia reflects a specific deficit in auditory sensory memory. The specificity of MMN deficits to schizophrenia remains controversial; some (but not all) studies have also reported a reduced MMN in association with depression.

The P300

The P300 is probably the best-studied of all ERP components, both in healthy volunteers and in psychiatric populations. The standard paradigm eliciting the P300 is similar to the one described above in relation to the MMN: a series of events are presented of which one class is rarer than the other—hence the name *oddball task.* Subjects are required to respond in some way to the rarer of the two events. The ERP elicited consists of a positive deflection that is maximal over the parietal/central scalp electrodes and has a latency of at least 300 msec and as much as 900 msec. In simple oddball tasks, the amplitude of the P300 depends on probability: the rarer the event, the larger the P300. It has been proposed that the P300 reflects the process by which contextual information is updated within memory. Several investigators, however, have noted that the P300 does not appear to be a unitary component. Indeed, recent fMRI studies that used oddball paradigms revealed widespread brain activation, distributed throughout many cortical and subcortical regions.

There have been numerous investigations of the P300 in patients with a variety of psychiatric disorders, particularly schizophrenia. The most robust finding in schizophrenia patients is of an abnormally reduced P300 amplitude. In some studies, the P300 latency is increased. The reduced P300 amplitude is particularly robust when auditory rather than visual stimuli are presented. The reduced P300 amplitude has been described in patients having their first episode of psychosis and in patients who are not taking medication. Some studies have suggested that the reduced P300 amplitude is associated with negative symptoms and with positive thought disorder (disorganized speech). Moreover, there is some evidence that the P300 amplitude becomes larger as symptoms ameliorate in the same patients over time, although it does not appear to normalize completely. These findings suggest that the reduced P300 may be both a state and a trait marker in schizophrenia.

A reduced P300 has also been reported in individuals who are at risk for developing schizophrenia and in healthy individuals who have loosening of associations similar to that observed in schizophrenia patients with positive thought disorder. Some studies, but not all, have reported a greater reduction of the P300 amplitude on the left than the right side in schizophrenia. Several studies also have linked structural gray matter deficits in temporal regions with a reduced P300 in schizophrenia.

Although an abnormal P300 is a very reliable finding in schizophrenia, it is not specific to schizophrenia. Studies have also reported abnormalities in the P300 waveform in association with dementia, substance abuse, depression, anxiety disorders (panic disorder, obsessive-compulsive disorder, and posttraumatic stress disorder) and in association with some personality disorders (schizoid, antisocial, and borderline).

The N400

The N400 ERP component is a negative shift in the ERP waveform that occurs approximately 400 msec following the onset of contextually inappropriate words. The N400 was first described in association with conceptual (i.e., semantic and pragmatic) violations in sentences (e.g., the N400 elicited in response to the word "dog" is of greater amplitude than the N400 elicited to the word "milk" when preceded by the sentence fragment, "He took coffee with sugar and ___"). Subsequent studies have established that the N400 amplitude is sensitive to the organization of semantic memory during the processing of word pairs, whole sentences, and whole discourse.

The observation that many patients with schizophrenia appear to show abnormalities in processing relationships between concepts provided the impetus for a large number of studies that have examined the N400 in schizophrenia. Some of these studies report a relatively intact N400 congruity effect in schizophrenia. Other studies, however, have reported an abnormally reduced N400 effect in both sentence and word-pair paradigms. One reason for these contradictory findings may be heterogeneity in the schizophrenia patient samples studied. Indeed, there is some evidence that the N400 effect is inversely correlated with severity of positive thought disorder in schizophrenia. Some investigators have also reported an increase in the absolute amplitude of the N400 waveform elicited in response to contextually appropriate and contextually inappropriate words, suggesting that schizophrenia patients have difficulty processing the meaning of words, regardless of the surrounding context.

Modifications of standard word association and sentence anomaly paradigms have yielded additional insights into the nature of conceptual abnormalities in schizophrenia. In a "mediated semantic priming" paradigm, an N400 congruity effect to words such as "stripes" preceded by indirectly related words such as "lion" (related to "tiger," which in turn is related to "stripes") has been reported in schizophrenia patients but not healthy control subjects. This finding is consistent with the hypothesis that activity spreads abnormally far across interconnected representations in semantic memory in schizophrenia patients. In a sentence paradigm, an N400 effect was elicited in healthy volunteers, but not in patients with schizophrenia, in response to words (e.g., "river") that were preceded by a semantically associated homonym (e.g., "bridge") when the surrounding context (e.g., "They took out their cards and started to play ___") suggested the secondary meaning of the homonym. Whereas in control subjects, the context of the whole sentence overrode the semantic associative effects of the sentence's individual words, this result did not occur in patients with schizophrenia.

Probably the most robust abnormality described across N400 studies in schizophrenia is an increased N400 latency. This abnormality has been reported in both word and sentence paradigms and suggests that the contextual integration of words may be delayed in schizophrenia.

Extracting Spatial Information: Source Localization From Multichannel Encephalography and Magnetoencephalography

The high temporal resolution of electrophysiological techniques is a clear advantage over other functional neuroimaging techniques—such as fMRI, positron emission tomography (PET), and single photon emission computed tomography (SPECT)—that look at events over the course of seconds. However, the EEG and ERPs provide very little information about the anatomic location of the neural systems that give rise to scalp-recorded voltage patterns.

In the past few years, there has been some progress toward improving the spatial resolution of EEG/ERPs by measuring over multiple channels distributed across the scalp surface and by using source localization methods to locate the underlying neural generator(s). In parallel, another technique—magnetoencephalography—has evolved from single-channel systems to multichannel systems that can monitor well over 100 channels simultaneously. The magnetoencephalogram (MEG) detects a magnetic signal that is derived from the same electrical currents that produce the EEG. Indeed, the raw MEG strikingly resembles the EEG, with alpha, mu, and tau rhythms. Similarly, the same types of signal averaging as described above that give rise to distinct ERP components also give rise to analogous waveforms when similar paradigms are used in the MEG (Figure 6–4). However, rather than focusing on the waveform itself, most MEG studies have emphasized source localization.

In the following section, I introduce the principles of source localization. I highlight implications of dif-

ferences in the EEG and MEG signals and emphasize some caveats in regard to interpreting source localization data. I then summarize the potential for such methods to yield new insights into psychiatric disorders.

Source Localization

Multichannel electroencephalography and magnetoencephalography can be used to generate spatial maps of the EEG potential and the magnetic field, respectively, over the surface of the scalp at different points in time. There are important differences in the types of maps derived from MEG and EEG. These differences can be predicted from magnetic and electrical theory and have important implications for determining the underlying source that gives rise to the two types of maps. First, for a source that is oriented radially with respect to the scalp surface (including sources near the center of the head), an EEG signal, but not a MEG signal, can be detected over the scalp. In other words, the EEG sees both radial and tangential sources, whereas the MEG sees only tangential sources. Second, for sources that are oriented tangentially to the scalp surface, because of the orthogonality between magnetic and electrical fields, the MEG map is perpendicular to the EEG map. Third, the electrical conduction of currents through the brain and skull leads to *smearing,* or low-pass filtering of the voltage pattern in EEG, whereas the MEG is only minimally affected by surface smearing. Therefore, the MEG produces a somewhat "tighter" map than the EEG. For all of these reasons, MEG and EEG recordings provide different but complementary information about underlying neural sources and are therefore often collected together.

A mathematical model can then be applied from maps at the scalp surface to estimate the most likely source in the brain responsible for this surface field distribution. For a single focal source (or dipole), this mathematical model is relatively straightforward and is called a simple "inverse solution." This model must take into account neurophysiological and neuroanatomic information. For example, one would not expect to localize primary sensory sources extracerebrally or in white matter distant from primary sensory cortex. One can then apply a "goodness of fit" calculation to reflect the agreement between the known surface topography that the estimated source would produce as a function of the ideal mathematical "forward solution" and the actually measured field pattern.

More complex mathematical models must be ap-

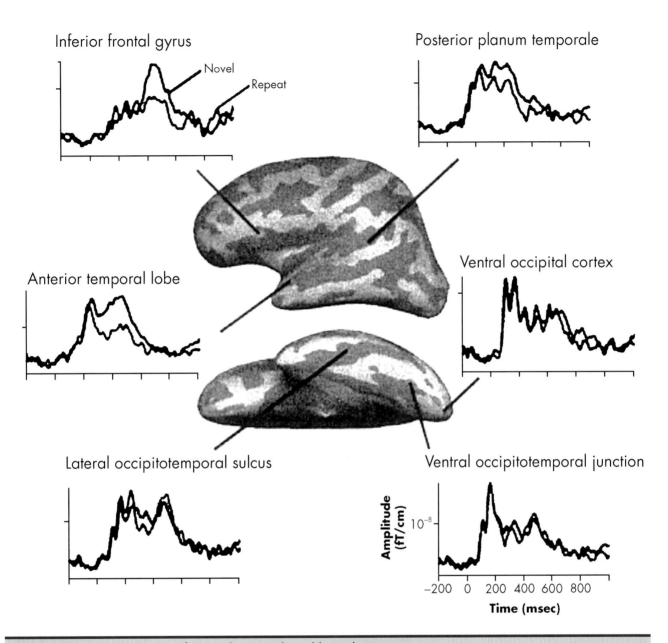

Figure 6–4.   Time courses of MEG data at selected brain locations.
Waveforms show activity in response to words that are novel or repeated during a word-stem completion task.
Occipital regions are activated early and do not change with repetition, whereas more anterior regions activate later
and show strong replication effects.
Source.   Reprinted from Dhond RP, Buckner RL, Dale AM, et al.: "Spatiotemporal Maps of Brain Activity Underlying Word Gen-
eration and Their Modification During Repetition Priming." *Journal of Neuroscience* 21(10):3564–3571, 2001. Copyright 2001, The
Society for Neuroscience. Used with permission.

plied to more complex maps. For example, longer-
latency endogenous complex potentials such as the
N400 probably arise from multiple anatomic sources. A
given spatiotemporal voltage pattern at the scalp may
arise from more than one configuration of sources and
is determined not only by their sites but also by their
orientations. Thus, even if it is mathematically possible
to calculate the inverse solution in such cases (and

sometimes even to find a relatively high goodness of
fit), it is important to recognize that this solution is not
necessarily correct. Nonetheless, the application of
such complex models has already yielded new insights
into the time course of brain activity during higher-
order cognitive processes such as memory and language (Figure 6–5).

One approach that has been employed to improve

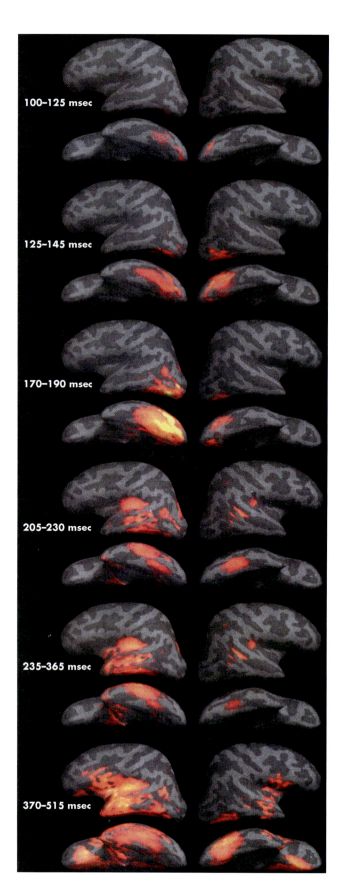

Figure 6–5. Estimated cortical activity patterns at different latencies after reading word stems, as measured with magnetoencephalography.

Activation begins with a bilateral visual response in the posterior occipital cortex (100–125 msec) and subsequently spreads forward into the ventral occipital cortex (125–145 msec) and lateralizes to the left hemisphere (170–190 msec). It then spreads to both posteroventral and lateral temporal areas (205–230 msec) and progressively extends to the anterior temporal (235–365 msec) and ventral prefrontal (370–515 msec) cortices, before fading after 515 msec.

Source. Reprinted from Dhond RP, Buckner RL, Dale AM, et al.: "Spatiotemporal Maps of Brain Activity Underlying Word Generation and Their Modification During Repetition Priming." *Journal of Neuroscience* 21(10):3564–3571, 2001. Copyright 2001, The Society for Neuroscience. Used with permission.

source modeling is to use fMRI data (collected by using identical stimulus presentation paradigms in the same subjects) as a spatial constraint. Important caveats apply to use of such an approach, however. Whereas the coupling between electrical activity in the brain and the EEG and MEG signals measured on the surface of the scalp follows from fundamental laws of physics and is relatively well understood, the coupling between neuronal activity and hemodynamic measures such as fMRI is not well understood. Thus, the precise relationships between hemodynamic signals measured with fMRI and electrical and magnetic signals measured with EEG and MEG are unclear. In particular, there are few quantitative data on how the magnitude of the hemodynamic response varies as a function of the amplitude and duration of electromagnetic activity. There is, however, increasing evidence for a strong degree of spatial correlation between various measures of local electrical activity and local hemodynamic signals. Some of the most persuasive evidence for such a correlation comes from a direct comparison of maps obtained through use of voltage-sensitive dyes, reflecting depolarization of neuronal membranes in superficial cortical layers, and maps derived from intrinsic optical signals, reflecting changes in light absorption due to changes in blood volume and oxygenation. Earlier animal studies have also shown strong correlations among local field potentials, spiking activity, and voltage-sensitive dye signals. Moreover, studies using invasive electrical recordings and fMRI to compare localization of functional activity in humans also provide evidence for a spatial correlation between the local electrophysiological response and the hemodynamic response.

Use of Magnetoencephalography in Psychiatry

The two current most common clinical uses of magnetoencephalography are in localization of epileptiform activity and presurgical mapping of sensory cortex prior to neurosurgical procedures.

The use of multichannel electroencephalography and magnetoencephalography in psychiatric research is in its infancy. Nonetheless, MEG studies have already contributed to our knowledge of specific components such as early auditory field potentials (the N100) in schizophrenia and somatosensory ERPs in affective psychoses. As discussed earlier, the development of more comprehensive models and the integration of magnetoencephalography with other functional neuroimaging techniques will enable study of the sources that give rise to endogenous ERPs. Such research will allow us to gain insight into the spatial and temporal dynamics of neural systems underlying abnormal cognitive function in psychiatric disorders.

Suggested Readings

EEG and qEEG

Hughes JR, John ER: Conventional and quantitative electroencephalography in psychiatry. J Neuropsychiatry Clin Neurosci 11:190–208, 1999

Introduction to ERPs

Rugg MD, Coles MGH: Electrophysiology of Mind: Event-Related Brain Potentials and Cognition (Oxford Psychology Series, No. 25). Oxford, UK, Oxford University Press, 1997

The P300

Donchin E, Coles MGH: Is the P300 component a manifestation of context updating? Behavioral and Brain Science 11:355–372, 1988

Ford JM: Schizophrenia: the broken P300 and beyond. Psychophysiology 36(6):667–682, 1999

The N400

Kutas M, Van Petten C: Event-related brain potential studies of language, in Advances in Psychophysiology: A Research Annual: 1988, Vol 3. Edited by Ackles PK, Jennings JR, Coles MGH. Greenwich, CT, JAI Press, 1988, pp 129–187

Sitnikova T, Salisbury DF, Kuperberg G, et al: Electrophysiological insights into language processing in schizophrenia. Psychophysiology 39:851–860, 2002

MEG and Combined MEG–fMRI Data

Dale AM, Liu AK, Fischl BR, et al: Dynamic statistical parametric mapping: combining fMRI and MEG for high-resolution imaging of cortical activity. Neuron 26:55–67, 2000

Hari R, Levanen S, Raij T: Timing of human cortical functions during cognition: role of MEG. Trends Cogn Sci 4:455–462, 2000

Reite M, Teale P, Rojas DC: Magnetoencephalography: applications in psychiatry. Biol Psychiatry 45:1553–1563, 1999

7

Neuroimaging in Psychiatric Practice

What Might the Future Hold?

Scott L. Rauch, M.D.

It is exciting to consider the future of medical science. In the case of neuroimaging in psychiatry, numerous ongoing developments suggest that the future of our field will be most exciting indeed. In this chapter, I discuss some relevant recent technological advances in neuroimaging and their implications for clinical psychiatry; moreover, I speculate about additional innovations, emphasizing potential clinical as well as research applications.

New and Emerging Neuroimaging Techniques

Throughout this volume, the individual chapters are replete with descriptions of modern imaging techniques. In several instances, emerging technology has also been described. In this section, I attempt to provide an overview of the emerging imaging techniques and how they might influence the field.

Spiral Computed Tomography

Within the realm of structural neuroimaging, spiral computed tomography (CT) represents an innovation that allows high-quality CT images to be obtained with shorter acquisition times. In conventional CT, slices are acquired one at a time as the X-ray beam source makes one full revolution around the body. With spiral CT, multiple slices are acquired with each revolution of the X-ray beam source as the body is advanced through the bore of the gantry. Hence, as the name suggests, the X-ray beam follows a spiral pattern in relation to the body. Essentially, innovations in hardware and image analysis support this new modality by providing high-quality reconstructions despite more limited sampling. Shorter acquisition time may be of particular relevance in psychiatry; to the extent that patients with disturbed mental status (e.g., agitation, psychosis) may have difficulty cooperating with or remaining still during scanning procedures, rapid image acquisition is of great benefit. Furthermore, spiral CT enables extension of conventional CT applications to include CT fluoroscopy. Although

CT fluoroscopy is not of immediate relevance to psychiatry, the trend toward improved temporal resolution and the potential for functional applications with CT may herald future psychiatric applications in this domain as well. It should be kept in mind that the earliest functional magnetic resonance imaging (MRI) methods entailed the use of contrast in conjunction with structural MRI at sufficient temporal resolution to visualize correlates of blood flow as an index of brain function.

Diffusion Imaging

Diffusion imaging refers to a family of MRI-based techniques that have the capacity to measure indices reflecting the diffusion of water within brain tissue. One type of diffusion imaging, called either diffusion tensor imaging (DTI) or diffusion tensor MRI (DT-MRI), exploits the fact that water molecules diffuse at different rates and in different directions, depending on the orientation of fiber bundles. More specifically, water diffuses more readily in parallel to the orientation of fiber bundles and less readily perpendicular to the orientation of fiber bundles. Consequently, using DT-MRI methods, researchers are now able to map the orientation of white matter tracts in vivo. Although still in its infancy, this method promises to be very powerful for delineating white matter abnormalities in psychiatric and neurological disorders, as well as in neurosurgical contexts. DT-MRI is especially promising as a tool for investigating what might be abnormalities of connectivity among brain regions. For developmental neuropsychiatric disorders, such techniques may reveal abnormalities that provide a substrate for imaging-based diagnostic procedures in psychiatry.

Diffusion-weighted imaging (DWI) can also provide information that is relevant to the viability of brain tissue, because certain pathological processes alter the local diffusion constant. DWI has recently been shown to reveal loci of acute and evolving stroke. This represents an innovation with tremendous potential ramifications for clinical neurology and psychiatry. Although conventional MRI and CT have long provided means for assessing infarcts that are several days old, DWI now enables clinicians to visualize strokes in evolution or only several hours old.

Magnetoencephalography, Electroencephalography, and Functional MRI

Magnetoencephalography (MEG) exploits the magnetic influence of electrical transmission within the brain to measure indices of brain activity at high temporal resolution. MEG has several limitations and at present is primarily reserved for research applications. For instance, MEG is sensitive only to brain activity near the surface. Furthermore, until recently, spatial localization with MEG was quite poor. However, new advances combining MEG with functional MRI (fMRI) have led to a capacity for visualizing surface brain activity with excellent temporal resolution (by MEG) and superior spatial localization (thanks to data from fMRI). Analogous strategies have also been used to combine data from electroencephalography (EEG) and fMRI. Use of such techniques opens the door to an entirely new brand of functional imaging in which movies, rather than still pictures, can be produced to illustrate regional cortical activity in real time. It is the hope of investigators that these temporo-spatial brain activity maps will provide unparalleled power for characterizing cortical brain activity patterns—adding the dimension of time to the three dimensions of space. Thus, MEG (or EEG), together with fMRI, might enable a much richer data set upon which to base discriminations among psychiatric, neurological, and medical conditions. Therefore, these new techniques represent a very promising potential for future advances in imaging-based diagnosis in psychiatry.

Optical Imaging

Optical imaging relies on the physical properties of light and its interaction with the brain and cerebral vasculature to create images of brain structure or function. Among the wide array of new and emerging optical imaging methods, so-called near-infrared spectroscopy (NIRS) and diffuse optical tomography (DOT) are of particular relevance to psychiatry. NIRS and DOT allow noninvasive in vivo measurement of regional brain activation by means of transmission of light. Somewhat analogous to concepts that enabled the advent of noncontrast fMRI, functional optical imaging relies on differences in the light-absorbing properties of oxyhemoglobin and deoxyhemoglobin to characterize regional brain activation. In fact, whereas fMRI indirectly measures changes in deoxyhemoglobin, NIRS is capable of separately quantifying these two hemoglobin species. NIRS is comparable in sensitivity to fMRI and actually has several advantages over other functional imaging modalities: low cost, potential for portability, and—given that neither ionizing radiation nor a high magnetic field environment are required—minimal risks or contraindications. The principal disadvantages of NIRS in comparison with fMRI include shallow penetration depth and absence of a tandem capacity to characterize brain structure for anatomic reference. It should be noted that this is a very active area of research; optical imaging methods may also be refined to provide techniques for absolute quantification of neuronal metabolism as well as hemodynamic changes. Practically, there is great excitement about optical imaging in psychiatry, because it promises to enable in vivo studies of central nervous system activity in infants and very young children that might otherwise be impossible. Furthermore, because of optical imaging's portability and tolerance of subject movement, in situ studies of plasticity, such as during learning and/or rehabilitation, and the capturing of events in their natural settings, such as the tics of Tourette's disorder or interventions such as exposure therapy, will become feasible. Finally, there is interest in developing these techniques to enable low-cost, portable brain imaging in the context of space travel and other special circumstances, such as in emergency response vehicles.

Summary of New Imaging Techniques

Together, these new techniques offer a revolutionary array of methods for investigating and characterizing brain structure and function. Ultimately, it is an empirical matter as to which of these will provide clinically useful information to aid with diagnosis and/or treatment of psychiatric conditions. Judging from recent work in the field, it is reasonable to predict that valuable contributions to our understanding of psychiatric disease and its pathophysiology will follow from integrating these various approaches in a complementary or synergistic manner. In the next section, I shift to consider how currently available imaging methods can be applied to support future advances in psychiatry.

New Applications of Existing Imaging Techniques in Psychiatry

Psychiatric neuroimaging research is still a relatively new field. Hence, investigators in this arena are still discovering and refining new strategies for applying neuroimaging tools. "Translational research" refers to the body of studies designed to translate more basic scientific information into a form that can be used in clinical practice. In the case of psychiatric neuroimag-

ing, there are now several strategies that allow investigators to begin bridging the gap between research and clinical practice. In this section, I discuss emerging strategies for applying contemporary imaging tools to enhance diagnosis and treatment selection in psychiatry.

Enhanced Diagnosis and Extended Phenotypes

Conventional structural neuroimaging techniques have long been used in psychiatric practice to rule in or rule out general medical causes of disturbed mental status. However, the field continues to await legitimate and established applications to guide clinical assessment of patients with psychiatric disorders. Here it is instructive to reflect upon the fundamental purpose of diagnosis in clinical medicine. In general, diagnostic schemes are designed to serve an organizing function, to furnish a basis for explanations, and to provide predictive information about natural course as well as response to various treatments. Armed with such information, patients and their families, along with their doctors, can be informed about what to expect and can also obtain guidance with respect to which courses of action—including selection of treatments—will produce which outcomes.

One of the great problems in psychiatry, unlike many other subspecialties of medicine, is that the diagnostic scheme currently established in our field is not well grounded in known pathophysiology, principally because the pathophysiology of psychiatric disorders is not yet understood. Consequently, in contrast to the medical model, psychiatry's current diagnostic entities are syndromes (i.e., characteristic constellations of signs and symptoms) rather than diseases per se (i.e., conditions reflecting a specific pathophysiological or disease process). In fact, one of the important challenges facing psychiatry today is to refine our diagnostic scheme so that it better reflects underlying pathophysiology.

The science of developing and improving diagnostic tests in medicine relies on the existence of a "gold standard" method for determining diagnosis in the first place. This fact underscores the limitation we face in psychiatry, where we lack a pathophysiology-based nosology. For us, the current gold standard of a clinical diagnosis cannot serve as the basis for judging the absolute quality of diagnostic information from other sources, such as neuroimaging or genetics, if we suspect that these more direct measures of pathophysiology will ultimately constitute the gold standard.

Predictive validity is one yardstick that can be used to measure even a gold standard method of diagnosis. In fact, early diagnosis—before an individual develops all of the signs and symptoms of a condition—can be of great clinical value. In Alzheimer's disease (AD), for instance, there has been great interest in developing a means for early diagnosis so that treatments designed to slow the progression of the disease can be initiated as early as possible. In the case of AD, methods have been developed for combining data from many sources to make the diagnosis with high specificity and sensitivity before the full constellation of clinical signs and symptoms have evolved. Some of the most powerful strategies for early diagnosis of AD entail use of data from functional and structural neuroimaging tests in conjunction with neuropsychological data. But how do clinical investigators in this area determine the accuracy of such predictive diagnoses? Each patient must be followed longitudinally 1) to determine how the clinical signs and symptoms evolve over successive years of life and 2) to examine the neuropathological profile within the brain after death. Thus, in the case of AD, whereas the syndrome as defined by clinical assessment serves as a short-term gold standard, the fact that this disease has a defining appearance by neuropathological examination at autopsy provides an ultimate gold standard.

In the case of primary psychiatric disorders, there are several areas in which we might envision developing neuroimaging tests of early diagnosis that could be of substantial clinical value. For example, it might be useful at presentation of schizotypal traits to be able to predict which subjects would progress to schizophrenia. Likewise, it would be useful to be able to assess patients at the time of an initial major depressive episode to accurately predict which ones were at increased vulnerability for future manic episodes (i.e., distinguishing unipolar from bipolar disease). This direction of psychiatric neuroimaging research may have great potential but has remained largely unexplored to date. The idea of being able to test children to determine their vulnerability to development of various disorders later in life is somewhat more controversial.

In fact, many investigators believe that the best predictors of natural course in psychiatry will entail the combination of genetic and neuroimaging information. After all, it is likely that neuroimaging data provide the most direct and comprehensive information regarding the anatomic, chemical, and physiological state of the human brain in vivo. Moreover, by using various challenge paradigms (e.g., pharmacological and cognitive challenges) dynamic aspects of these functions can be ascertained across various contexts. In a complementary fashion, an individual's genotype provides the ultimate information regarding his or her intrinsic programmed vulnerabilities as well as resilience factors.

Interestingly, advances in psychiatric genetics require refined definitions of phenotypes: "phenotype" refers to the external appearance, clinical presentation, or net outward manifestation of the genotype. So-called extended phenotypes (or endophenotypes) refer to the concept of using internal anatomic or physiological measures (e.g., brain-imaging profiles) to define the phenotype.

In the future, it is anticipated that use of multimodal imaging techniques—perhaps in conjunction with other indices, such as genetic assessments—will lead to early diagnosis of psychiatric conditions or associated risk factors. In an iterative manner, identifying specific brain-imaging profiles that predict the natural course of illness will facilitate the development of a pathophysiology-based diagnostic scheme in psychiatry. Furthermore, by providing extended phenotypes, brain imaging will help advance psychiatric genetics.

Predictors of Treatment Response

Beyond enhanced diagnosis and predictors of natural course, brain-imaging profiles can also be used to predict treatment response. There is already a growing literature describing results of initial longitudinal studies that have identified possible predictors of response to various treatments for psychiatric diseases. The typical paradigm entails gathering brain-imaging data from a group of subjects prior to their entry into a treatment trial. At the end of the treatment trial, once the subjects' respective outcomes are known, these measures of response can be correlated with aspects of the pretreatment brain-imaging profile. Thus, investigators are able to identify which characteristics within the pretreatment brain-imaging profile predict subsequent good or poor outcome in response to the specific treatment. This application of neuroimaging in psychiatry is an exciting one, as it promises a means for predicting, for a given patient, the likelihood of a good or poor response to any of a range of possible treatments. In this way, we can envision neuroimaging tests to guide selection among psychiatric treatments. Although such tests may rarely be cost-effective for choosing between medications or psychotherapies, one could imagine them being of great clinical value when considering treatments of relatively higher risk or higher cost, such as electroconvulsive therapy or neurosurgery.

Neurochemical Methods to Monitor Treatment

Neurochemical imaging techniques provide methods for monitoring treatment, especially with regard to psychotropic medications. Already, magnetic resonance spectroscopy (MRS) has been used to measure the cerebral concentration of specific MRS-visible medications, such as lithium or fluoxetine. It has become clear that for some patients, relatively low or relatively high brain concentrations of medication are achieved with standard dosages. In the future, such tests of chemical concentrations within the brain may be helpful in titrating dosages of psychotropic medications. Furthermore, it may ultimately become possible to target specific brain regions for enhanced concentration or activity of medications—for example, by causing regional changes in blood–brain barrier permeability or by administering precursor medications that require activation in situ. Similarly, receptor characterization studies—consisting of positron emission tomography (PET) or single photon emission computed tomography (SPECT) in conjunction with radioactively labeled tracers—can be used to characterize receptor affinity, density/number, and occupancy. Such methods may become clinically useful in identifying whether a given patient is receiving a sufficient dosage of a medication.

Summary of New Applications of Existing Imaging Techniques

New paradigms incorporating existing imaging methods promise to advance the development of our diagnostic scheme in psychiatry. Furthermore, neuroimaging methods will progressively be applied to make early diagnoses and to predict the natural course of psychiatric disease. Finally, neuroimaging tools may soon be used in the clinical setting to predict treatment response as well as monitor treatment to optimize therapy for psychiatric patients.

Development of New Treatments Guided by Neuroimaging

New Psychotropic Agents

Though many of the classic psychotropic agents were serendipitously found to be effective as treatments for psychiatric disorders, we are now in an age in which new psychiatric drug development is proceeding more systematically and rationally. As candidate medications are synthesized or discovered, several crucial steps must be taken before progressing to large-scale studies of efficacy in humans. Following animal studies of safety, pharmacokinetics, and pharmacological effects, it is often useful to characterize the pharmacokinetics and pharmacodynamics of these agents in human subjects. In fact, functional imaging techniques (e.g., PET) can be used to quantify the distribution of radiolabeled forms of these compounds throughout the body. For certain agents that may disproportionately collect in specific organs, drug distribution becomes a critically important consideration with respect to possible toxicities. Also, by using radiolabeled forms of the candidate compound, investigators are able to quantify its regional distribution within the brain as well as its binding profile in situ. Alternatively, investigators sometimes use specific well-characterized radiolabeled tracers in conjunction with unlabeled forms of candidate medications to indirectly measure the effects of the candidate agent (i.e., by measuring how the candidate agent "competes" with the well-understood compound for binding to receptor sites). This indirect strategy is used in cases where it might be difficult to radioactively label the candidate medication or when there is concern that the labeling process might alter the pharmacological action of the candidate medication. Perhaps surprisingly, in vitro studies of binding properties often yield only poor approximations of how such candidate medications actually behave in the brains of living, breathing humans. Hence, these in vivo brain-imaging methods have become a very important and valuable part of the drug discovery process, particularly for medications that target the central nervous system.

Advances in Neurosurgical Treatment and Brain Stimulation

Neurosurgical treatment for psychiatric diseases has a long and controversial history. Since the 1980s, there have been important advances in this field, in terms of both the surgical methods applied and the systematic manner in which clinical data have been collected. Extant data now indicate that several of these procedures have modest efficacy and acceptable risks for the treatment of individuals with severe, otherwise treatment-refractory obsessive-compulsive disorder (OCD) or major depression. Currently, the best-studied and best-accepted operations are anterior cingulotomy, anterior capsulotomy, and limbic leucotomy. The advent of stereotactic functional neurosurgery helped to refine the reliability of lesion placement. Likewise, the advent of radiosurgical methods, with the gamma knife, led to investigation of ablative procedures (i.e., anterior capsulotomy) performed without the need for craniotomy. Finally, ongoing research, still in an early stage, is being conducted to investigate the application of deep brain stimulation (DBS) as a treatment for OCD or depression. In comparison with ablative procedures, DBS offers the obvious advantages of more flexibility and reversibility.

In several respects, neuroimaging plays an important role in this area. First, structural MRI is used to plan and confirm the placement of lesions (in the case of the ablative procedures) or the stimulation electrodes (in the case of DBS). Second, investigators have begun to conduct neuroimaging studies to identify predictors of treatment response and also to establish the structural and functional consequences of these procedures. Pretreatment imaging data paired with acute postoperative and long-term follow-up imaging data can be used to explore the changes associated with effective versus ineffective interventions. In this way, it is hoped that knowledge will be gained about the mechanism of action by which these treatments exert their effects—both beneficial and adverse.

Third, there is much interest in the idea of using imaging data to tailor the specific application of these methods to individual patients. For example, in the case of DBS, functional brain-imaging data gathered during acute stimulation, using various stimulation parameters, might one day be used to guide clinicians in selecting treatment settings. Likewise, in the case of ablative neurosurgical treatments, it is conceivable that the precise lesion site could be individually tailored on the basis of results from a presurgical functional imaging test.

In addition to surgical interventions, including ablative procedures and DBS, the technique of transcranial magnetic stimulation (TMS) provides a means for relatively noninvasive regional brain stimulation. Investigators have recently begun to explore potential clinical applications of TMS in the treatment of OCD and depression. More generally, it is appealing to consider that manipulation of focal brain activity may offer a way to treat some psychiatric diseases. In its current form, TMS can be used to facilitate or inhibit regional cortical activity. Consequently, one might imagine that TMS would be a potential treatment for psychiatric disorders with known regional cortical dysfunction.

Much as in the case of surgical treatments, imaging may conceivably play a role in TMS-based therapies by enabling 1) enhanced placement to match a specific targeted location, 2) prediction of treatment response, and 3) individual tailoring of treatment through provision of a) pretreatment guidance regarding optimal targeting and b) ongoing information to optimize stimulation parameters on the basis of the individual's brain response.

Conclusions

The future of psychiatric neuroimaging is bright. In addition to having a continuing tremendous role in psychiatric research, neuroimaging is likely to progressively play a prominent role in the clinical psychiatric setting. New imaging techniques will expand the range of parameters we can measure while extending the boundaries of temporal and spatial resolution and overcoming other obstacles. It is plausible that the near future will see us able to quantitatively assess numerous indices of brain structure, function, and chemistry in real time, safely, in patients of essentially any age, while awake and, in some instances, freely moving. The new gamut of imaging technologies combined with innovative paradigms will soon support advances toward early diagnosis and predictors of both natural illness course and treatment response. As neuroimaging and genetic research progress in parallel, it is likely that we will witness an evolution of the psychiatric diagnostic scheme toward one that is better grounded in the pathophysiological basis of disease. Finally, psychiatric neuroimaging techniques will play a central role in the development of new and better treatments. This will include a role in the process of drug development and also in the fields of neurosurgical treatment and brain stimulation. These capabilities promise to revolutionize the practice of psychiatry during the current century.

Suggested Readings

Bonmassar G, Schwartz DP, Liu AK, et al: Spatiotemporal brain imaging of visual-evoked activity using interleaved EEG and fMRI recordings. Neuroimage 13:1035–1043, 2001

Cosyns P, Gabriels L, Nuttin B: Deep brain stimulation in severe treatment refractory OCD. Eur Psychiatry 17 (suppl 1): 31–32, 2002

Dougherty DD, Rauch SL (eds): Psychiatric Neuroimaging Research: Contemporary Strategies. Washington, DC, American Psychiatric Publishing, 2001

Frostig RD (ed): In Vivo Optical Imaging of Brain Function. New York, CRC Press, 2002

George MS, Belmaker RH (eds): Transcranial Magnetic Stimulation in Neuropsychiatry. Washington, DC, American Psychiatric Press, 2002

Hariri AR, Mattay VS, Tessitore A, et al: Serotonin transporter genetic variation and the response of the human amygdala. Science 297:400–403, 2002

Jobst KA, Barnetson LP, Shepstone BJ: Accurate prediction of histologically confirmed Alzheimer's disease and the differential diagnosis of dementia: the use of NINCDS-ADRDA and DSM-III-R criteria, SPECT, x-ray CT, and Apo E4 in medial temporal lobe dementias. Oxford Project to Investigate Memory and Aging. Int Psychogeriatr 10:271–302, 1998

Makris N, Rauch SL, Kennedy DN (eds): Diffusion imaging: principles, methods, and applications. CNS Spectrums 7(7), 2002

Rauch SL: Preparing for psychiatry in the 21st century, in Psychiatry: Update and Board Preparation. Edited by Stern TA, Herman JB. New York, McGraw-Hill, 2000, pp 579–583

Rauch SL, Dougherty DD, Cosgrove GR, et al: Cerebral metabolic correlates as potential predictors of response to anterior cingulotomy for obsessive compulsive disorder. Biol Psychiatry 50:659–667, 2001

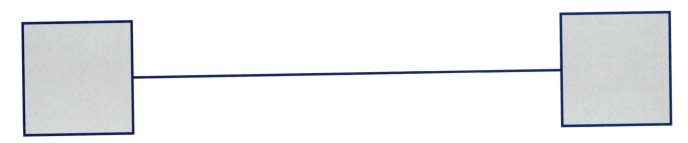

Index

*Page numbers printed in **boldface** type refer to tables or figures.*

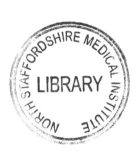